SHORT CASES FOR THE
PAEDIATRIC MEMBERSHIP

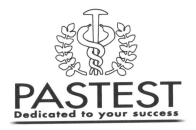

PASTEST

Dedicated to your success

SHORT CASES FOR THE PAEDIATRIC MEMBERSHIP

DR R M BEATTIE
Consultant Paediatrician

DR A T CLARK
Specialist Registrar

DR A L SMITH
Specialist Registrar

**Department of Paediatrics,
Peterborough District Hospital,
Peterborough**

First published 1999

ISBN 1 901198 25 1

A catalogue record for this book is available from the British Library.

Text prepared by Breeze Limited, Manchester.
Printed by Bell & Bain Ltd, Glasgow.

CONTENTS

INTRODUCTION

This book is intended to help with the MRCPCH Part Two clinical examination. It is not a complete textbook of paediatrics or a textbook of clinical examination, but a summary text of important information which will help with the examination. It has been put together to reflect commonly asked questions and short case scenarios with the help of over 60 candidates during the last 3–4 years who have written directly to me with details of their own experiences. It is supplemented by my own experience of teaching on membership courses.

The book is primarily about the short cases as this is the part of the exam candidates find most difficult and most often fail. Notes on the long case and viva examination are included at the back. The short cases are system specific and include notes on examination technique, useful background information and summaries of cases that have been seen in past exams.

The lists in this book are not exhaustive and focus on common and better known items rather than rarities. This is essential in your approach to answering questions, in order to avoid falling into black holes; for example when you mention a rare differential diagnosis and are asked to talk about it! All the conditions described in the text are frequently seen and a thorough knowledge of all of them is required.

Team up with a like-minded candidate; quiz each other and practice presenting to each other. Practice all parts of the exam. Although most candidates who fail do so on the short cases do not make the mistake of neglecting to practise all the parts of the exam as a significant number will fail either on the long case or the viva. Use the examples in the book.

Attend outpatients as this is where you will see many of the conditions which are likely to come up in the exam. Include visits to community clinics, the child development unit, audiology clinic and orthoptic clinic.

Remember that you may get a resuscitation scenario. A number of candidates have been shocked into failing when a resuscitation doll appears. This can be practised. Try to attend a PALS or APLS course and if not read the BMA produced APLS handbook (see Further Reading).

Many people have helped with this book. I have been assisted enormously by my co-authors Andrew Clark and Anne Smith who have enthusiastically discussed and helped write all aspects of this book and without whom I could not have produced it. I am grateful to Dr M Lal who contributed to the rheumatology and dermatology chapters. I would also like to acknowledge Drs Chan, Hyer, Rhodes and Maconochie who have read and commented on various sections.

I would finally like to acknowledge the many candidates who sent me details of their experiences in the exam, particularly those who attended the Ealing Paediatric courses which I have been fortunate to teach on and have provided much of my inspiration for this book.

R M Beattie
May 1999

PASTEST REVISION COURSES

Postgraduate medical exams have become increasingly competitive, don't let anyone be more prepared than you are. On a PasTest revision course you will experience outstanding tutors who teach in a lively and interactive way in order to focus your knowledge.

PasTest are the market leaders in MRCP revision courses. 25 years' experience allow us to:

- Select only the best lecturers in the field (and we continually assess their performance).
- Use teaching methods which are stimulating and make learning more enjoyable.
- Give you invaluable tips on exam preparation and presentation.

Consolidate your learning with a PasTest revision course, call now for details:

Freephone 0800 9809814

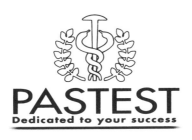

PasTest, Freepost, Knutsford, Cheshire WA16 7BR
Fax: 01565 650264
E-mail: enquiries@pastest.co.uk
Web site: http://www.pastest.co.uk

x

NOTES ON THE SHORT CASES

Many candidates fail because of the short cases. In many instances I am sure this is due to poor preparation regarding potential exam scenarios. Vital marks are lost because candidates do not know the answers to supplementary questions asked after the initial questions. For example, a candidate may be asked to look at a child's abdomen. In order to pass this short case the candidate needs to be able to examine the abdomen, know what he might find and be able to answer questions on what he finds. This means that more information than just how to carry out the examination is needed. Information is also required about potential conditions which may be encountered such as glycogen storage disorder, portal hypertension, thalassaemia or biliary atresia.

It is essential to be completely clear about how to examine any system. A personal method needs to be decided upon and learned. You will rapidly realise that there is no definitive way in which to examine any system. However, the examiner is unlikely to tolerate imprecise or clumsy clinical examination and this should be avoidable with proper preparation. You need to find your own scheme. Remember that the scenarios you meet may not be straightforward. This book suggests an examination scheme for most potential scenarios. You are also referred to standard texts of paediatric examination.

The differential diagnoses in this text are 'practical differential diagnoses' focusing particularly on common scenarios and ones which are likely to be seen in the exam. Many candidates report that they are not given the chance to present a full differential diagnosis, but are asked for one or two possibilities relating to the child that they have seen.

During the short case exam you will need to adopt an air of confidence about your findings and the way you present them, otherwise it will be easy for an examiner to sow doubt in your mind and throw you off balance. For example, a candidate was asked to examine an abdomen with bilateral masses and then asked to present her findings. She presented the patient as having an enlarged spleen and liver. The examiner was able to change the candidate's mind twice as to whether the masses were kidneys or liver and spleen in the subsequent discussion. Confidence in the exam comes from correct examination technique and relentless practice of examination and presentation. This should be in pairs or with a tutor. Team up with like-minded candidates who are doing the exam and practice with them.

Do not stop your examination when you have identified the organ in question. There is a set routine for examining an enlarged liver and you must continue with your examination until you are stopped. Another candidate was asked to examine the abdomen. There was an enlarged liver and the child had a fever, having just returned from Africa. The candidate correctly identified malaria as the diagnosis but failed the exam. On counselling she was told that her examination of the liver was inadequate because she did not percuss its size.

Furthermore, be confident about your findings. It is tempting to exclude a clear physical sign if you feel it does not fit in with the other signs. Another candidate was asked to examine the cardiovascular system and to comment afterwards. She correctly identified the missing left brachial pulse and the left thoracotomy scar, making the correct diagnosis of repaired aortic coarctation. However, this candidate also heard a soft ejection systolic murmur and could not fit it to the picture and so did not mention it. Of course, such a murmur is to be expected in coarctation. Despite this the candidate passed.

Finally, keep the momentum going. As long as you are moving you are earning points. Instead of stopping after you identify that a Mediterranean child has an enlarged spleen, say that the likely diagnosis is thalassaemia and that you would routinely check a full blood count, blood film and haemoglobin electrophoresis. If you don't you will probably be asked and this frustrates the examiners and wastes time. Fill in the gaps and move on to the next case.

BASIC FORMAT FOR CLINICAL EXAMINATION
- Introduce yourself to the child and parent
- Be prepared to talk about your findings as you proceed
- Observe
- Feel
- Auscultate
- Describe your findings
- Answer questions about your findings as you walk over to the next short case

Presentation skills are important and particularly the first few sentences you say about a certain scenario need to be practised. Examples of how to present cases are included in the subsequent chapters. You must practice short cases to excess before the exam. When presenting, it is useful to have a few general words which can be applied to most cases e.g. 'Harry is a boy who looks well grown and I would like to plot his weight on a centile chart...' This approach overcomes nerves and gives you time to compose yourself.

The information in this book is presented part in note form and part as it would appear in the exam using case scenarios to illustrate the knowledge required on a particular topic.

CHAPTER 1 – CARDIOLOGY

Cardiology short cases are a hard part of the exam. We have tried to give useful information and to highlight some of the important areas and more common topics covered. It is essential to have a good system of cardiovascular examination and some background knowledge to help with the interpretation of physical signs. In most short case scenarios it is sensible to talk your way through the examination of the case. In cardiovascular system examination however, particularly if the diagnosis is not obvious, then it is wise to keep your own counsel. Clearly, even if doing this, if you see something obvious e.g. Down's syndrome, cyanosis or chest wall scarring, it is wise to say so.

In addition to this chapter it is essential to read through paediatric cardiology in one of the standard texts.

SUMMARY
- ❑ Scheme for examination of the cardiovascular system
- ❑ Taking blood pressure
- ❑ Scars
- ❑ Heart sounds
- ❑ Murmurs
- ❑ Innocent murmurs
- ❑ Common associations of cardiac lesions
- ❑ Ventricular septal defect
- ❑ Atrial septal defect
- ❑ Pulmonary stenosis
- ❑ Aortic stenosis
- ❑ Coarctation of the aorta
- ❑ Dextrocardia
- ❑ The cyanosed child
- ❑ Fallot's tetralogy
- ❑ Complex congenital heart disease – post repair

SCHEME FOR EXAMINATION OF THE CARDIOVASCULAR SYSTEM

INSPECTION
- Dysmorphic features
- Failure to thrive
- Cyanosis
- Respiratory distress
- Harrison's sulci

Hands
- Clubbing
- Cyanosis

Pulse
- Brachial (babies), radial (older child)
- Peripheral pulses (may be best left to the end)
- Radiofemoral delay

Blood pressure
- Mention but don't necessarily do (but be prepared to if asked)

Face
- Anaemia
- Central cyanosis

Neck
- JVP (older child)

Scars
- Thoracotomy scars
- Median sternotomy scars

PALPATION
- Apex beat – including localisation, presence of heaves – check for dextrocardia
- Thrills – don't forget supra-sternal thrill and carotid thrill

AUSCULTATION

Listen in four areas
- Mitral (apex)
- Tricuspid (lower left sternal edge)
- Aortic (right second intercostal space)
- Pulmonary (left second intercostal space)

Several candidates have been asked to point out the areas to the examiner:
- The anatomical area may not be accurate e.g. aortic stenosis – see later
- Check for dextrocardia

Heart sounds
- Take note of these before assessing the nature of any murmur
- Are they present?
- Is the second heart sound normal?

Murmurs
- Timing in relation to cardiac cycle
- Systolic/diastolic/continuous/mixed systolic and diastolic – 'to and fro'
- Grade (I–VI)
- Site of maximal intensity, radiation (neck, axilla and back)
- Character
- Murmur enhancing moves – left lateral position, sitting forward

Grading of Murmurs

I	– barely audible
II	– medium intensity
III	– loud but no thrill
IV	– loud with a thrill
V	– very loud but still requires stethoscope to be on the chest
VI	– so loud, can be heard with stethoscope off the chest

FURTHER EXAMINATION

- Do not forget anything you may have left until the end e.g. blood pressure, femoral pulses
- Listen to the back for murmurs
- Palpate the liver

It is not unreasonable in a small child to move straight on to auscultation at the very beginning of the examination, if the patient is quiet, in order to listen to heart sounds and murmurs before the child becomes upset. It is probably best to explain yourself to the examiner if you perform the examination this way. Remember to complete the examination.

It is important to adapt your examination, if appropriate, and to be responsive to whatever the examiner asks. Clearly, if the examiner asks you to do cardiovascular examination then the full examination should be done. If you are asked to examine the heart then it is less clear. It is my view, although not a consensus view, that in this instance the full cardiovascular examination should be done unless the examiner specifically tells you to take short cuts. If the examiner asks you just to listen to the heart then that may be all he expects in that instance. If you are unclear what is expected of you, then it is perfectly reasonable to check with the examiner exactly what he wants.

TAKING BLOOD PRESSURE

You should know how to take blood pressure, as you may be asked to talk the examiner through the procedure or to take a blood pressure measurement.

Remember cuff width should be approximately 2/3rds of the length of the upper arm.

In neonates this may be difficult, and an estimate of systolic blood pressure can be obtained via the flush method.

- Apply the BP cuff, blanch the area distal to the cuff by squeezing/wrapping in an elastic bandage
- Inflate the cuff
- Release the pressure of the blanch
- Deflate the cuff slowly, the flushing corresponds to the approximate systolic pressure

In older children the auscultatory method is employed.

- Pick the appropriate cuff for the size of the arm
- Inflate the cuff whilst palpating the brachial/radial pulse until the pulse disappears
- Inflate the cuff a further 10 mmHg
- Place the stethoscope over the brachial artery
- Deflate the cuff slowly until regular sounds (the Korotkov's sounds) can just be heard through the stethoscope
- Note the systolic pressure as accurately as possible
- Continue to deflate the cuff slowly, the sounds get louder then suddenly become muffled and disappear
- Record the point at which the sounds become muffled as the diastolic pressure

Avoid cuffs that are too small as they may cause a falsely high BP.

In reality BP is often measured by a Doppler machine or dinamap. If you are not familiar with how to use these you should ask one of the nursing staff to teach you.

Approximate values for blood pressure in children	
Newborn	60 mmHg mean
Infancy	80/55 mmHg
Preschool	90/60 mmHg
School	100/65 mmHg

SCARS

It is important to note the presence of scars, especially the left thoracotomy scar, which is relatively common in exam cases, but may be difficult to see from the front.

If there are several scars this is also relevant e.g. thoracotomy scar (older scar) then central thoracotomy scar (later definitive procedure).

Causes of scars

Left thoracotomy	Right thoracotomy
• Shunt procedure	• Shunt procedure
• PDA ligation	• Tracheo-oesophageal fistula repair
• Coarctation repair	• Lung causes e.g. lobectomy
• Pulmonary artery banding	
• Lung causes e.g. lobectomy	

Sub mammary scar

• ASD

Central sternotomy scar

• Usually open heart surgery
• Any definitive procedure not covered by the above, both corrective and palliative

Corrective procedures

VSD repair, ASD repair, tetralogy of Fallot repair, arterial switch for repair of transposition of the great arteries.

Palliative procedures – temporary or permanent

• Central shunt procedures e.g. total cavo-pulmonary anastomoses
• Fontan
• Mustard, Senning
• Valve replacement

Other

• Lung or mediastinal surgery

HEART SOUNDS

First heart sound
(handwritten: closure of AV valves)

Loud when cardiac output high e.g. when nervous or excited, anaemia and pyrexia. Soft when low cardiac output or poor left ventricular function.

Second heart sound
(handwritten: Closure of AV & PV. aortic, pulmoary)

Important in the diagnosis of structural heart disease.

- Single or double – single if significant stenosis or atresia of arterial valve
- Split widely – atrial septal defect where the right ventricle is overfilled and pulmonary valve closure is delayed or mild pulmonary stenosis
- Fixed splitting – atrial septal defect, when there is no variation with respiration, the two atria are functioning as one and respiration has the same effect on both the pulmonary and systemic circulation
- Loud – e.g. pulmonary hypertension

Third heart sound

Rapid filling of the ventricles during diastole, present in 1/5th of all normal children. In cardiac failure a third sound may combine with other sounds to cause a gallop rhythm.

Fourth heart sound

This occurs shortly before the first heart sound, is almost always pathological but rare in children.

Ejection clicks

Classically occur in aortic valve and pulmonary valve stenosis, but may also be heard when there is a large dilated aorta in tetralogy of Fallot, coarctation of the aorta, patent ductus arteriosus or when there is a dilated pulmonary artery in pulmonary hypertension. The sound is made by the forceful opening of the valve.

Aortic click – lower left sternal edge and apex
Pulmonary click – second left intercostal space

MURMURS

Systolic murmurs

Can be functional (innocent) or pathological.

- Ejection systolic murmurs caused by forward flow of blood through an abnormal semilunar valve e.g. aortic stenosis, pulmonary stenosis
- Regurgitant murmurs caused by retrograde flow of blood through an incompetent atrioventricular valve e.g. mitral regurgitation (rare), tricuspid regurgitation (rare) or through a ventricular septal defect

Diastolic murmurs

Diastolic murmurs are always pathological and occur

- when the semilunar valves are incompetent – pulmonary regurgitation, aortic regurgitation
- when the atrioventricular valves are narrow – mitral stenosis
- when the valves are normal, but there is increased volume of blood flow through them, VSD = increased flow through the mitral valve, PDA = increased flow through the mitral valve

Causes of continuous murmurs

- Blalock-Taussig shunt
- AV malformation
- Aneurysm
- Collateral vessels
- Patent ductus arteriosus
- Venous hum
- Peripheral pulmonary stenosis
- Aortopulmonary window

INNOCENT MURMURS

INSTRUCTION

Examine this child's cardiovascular system

> **Case**
>
> *Jack is 4. He looks well and is thriving. There is no clubbing. His pulse and blood pressure are normal. There are no scars. His apex beat is normal and in the 5th left intercostal space. There are no heaves or thrills. There is a 2/6 ejection systolic murmur, maximal in the pulmonary area which does not radiate. The murmur is loudest when the child sits forward. The heart sounds are normal. CXR and ECG are normal.*

This is likely to be a pulmonary flow murmur.

NOTES ON INNOCENT MURMURS

Characteristics of an innocent murmur

- Localised
- Poorly conducting
- Musical/vibratory
- Soft grade 1–3/6
- Systolic
- Varies with posture
- Present in high output states, for example febrile illness
- Cardiac examination otherwise normal
- CXR, ECG normal

Pulmonary flow murmur

This is a very common murmur. Characteristically it is brief and in mid systole. It is loudest with the patient supine and during expiration. Occurs in children and adolescents of all ages and is commonly heard during hyperdynamic states such as fever.

$S_2 - Ⓝ$

L - II ICS

Still's murmur

Peak age 2–6, resolves towards adolescence. Grade 1–3 present in early systole, heart sounds normal. Maximum intensity lower left sternal edge. Vibratory. Best heard with the patient supine, reducing in intensity or disappearing when the patient sits up.

Venous hum

This is a continuous murmur most commonly heard in children aged 2–6 years. The diastolic component is usually loudest. It is best heard over the supraclavicular fossa on the right with the head turned to the other side. It may radiate and is often heard on both sides. There is sometimes an associated thrill. It disappears on lying flat or if the neck veins are compressed.

COMMON ASSOCIATIONS OF CARDIAC LESIONS

Down's syndrome
- Up to 50% are quoted to have some congenital heart defect
- Ventricular septal defects are the commonest lesions followed by atrioventricular septal defects
- PDA and tetralogy of Fallot are less common
- All children with Down's syndrome should be routinely sent for an echocardiogram
- Children with Down's syndrome develop pulmonary vascular disease earlier than other children, and hence with large cardiac defects will develop the Eisenmenger's complex at an earlier stage
- Be prepared to discuss the case of the Down's child with the complete AVSD. Decisions on medical versus surgical treatment, risks of operation, life expectancy etc. may be asked in your long case. Included in this part you may be asked to discuss the ethics of providing or withholding treatment.

Turner's syndrome (XO)
- Bicuspid aortic valve, usually non stenotic, in 1/3rd of patients
- Coarctation of aorta, less common but more serious

Noonan's syndrome (phenotypically like Turner's, without the chromosome defect)
- Pulmonary stenosis in a usually dysplastic valve, and hence not amenable to treatment by valvuloplasty
- ASD
- Cardiomyopathy

Williams' syndrome
- Supravalvular aortic stenosis
- Branch pulmonary artery stenosis

di George 22q deletion syndrome
- Aortic arch abnormalities
- Truncus arteriosus
- Pulmonary atresia and VSD

CHARGE association
- Fallot's tetralogy
- VSD
- AVSD
- Double outlet right ventricle

VACTERL association
- Fallot's tetralogy
- VSD

Infant of diabetic mother
- Hypertrophic cardiomyopathy
- VSD

Trisomy 18 – Edwards' syndrome
- VSD
- ASD
- PDA
- Coarctation of aorta
- Bicuspid aortic valve

Trisomy 13 – Patau's syndrome

- VSD
- ASD
- PDA
- Coarctation
- Bicuspid aortic valve

CHARGE association

This consists of
- Coloboma
- Heart disease
- Atresia choanae
- Retarded growth and development and/or CNS abnormalities
- Genital anomalies and/or hypogonadism
- Ear anomalies and/or deafness

VACTERL association, a non random association of malformations

This includes
- Vertebral defects
- Anal atresia
- Cardiac defects
- Tracheo-oesophageal fistula
- Renal defects
- Limb abnormalities.

This is an updated version of the **VATER** association.

VENTRICULAR SEPTAL DEFECT

This is one of the commonest short cases.

INSTRUCTION

Examine this child's cardiovascular system

INSPECTION

- Normal, patient appears well
- No tachypnoea or tachycardia

Hands

- No clubbing/cyanosis
- Pulses normal

Blood pressure

- Normal

Normal face

No scars

PALPATION

- Active precordium with thrill, normally at the left sternal edge

AUSCULTATION

- Loud, pansystolic murmur, maximal at the left sternal edge
- Grade IV
- No radiation, but heard all over the chest wall
- Second heart sound normal

Diagnosis: ventricular septal defect – haemodynamically insignificant.

Notes

- If the second heart sound is loud this suggests a large shunt and that there is pulmonary hypertension.
- If the second heart sound is loud it suggests elevated pulmonary arterial pressure, i.e. a haemodynamically significant VSD, therefore must mention the second heart sound
- If there is cardiomegaly and a diastolic rumble at the apex then the clinical features of heart failure are present implying a large defect with a significant shunt

Supplementary questions frequently asked

- How would you confirm this is a VSD?
- How would you follow this child up?
- What advice would you give the parents?
- Give the options for management
- What are the indications for surgery?
- How would you differentiate between VSD and innocent murmur?

NOTES ON VENTRICULOSEPTAL DEFECTS

Ventriculoseptal defects are the commonest congenital heart defects (30%). Defects usually occur in the membranous part of the septum with extension into the muscular septum, the so-called perimembranous VSD, although they may occur anywhere. The main haemodynamic effect is left ventricular volume overload and increased pulmonary blood flow. There is often a misconception that the right ventricle is overloaded due to the left to right shunt of blood. When the blood is being shunted in systole, the right ventricle is ejecting blood into the pulmonary artery, thus the blood is shunted directly into the pulmonary artery and hence into the lungs. This then returns to load the left ventricle during diastole.

Investigations

ECG, CXR, echocardiogram – 2 dimensional with colour flow Doppler. The latter is useful to help estimate the size of the shunt by examining the degree of volume overload of the left atrium and left ventricle. Cardiac catheterisation is not usually required.

In a small defect where the shunt is insignificant, there is usually no haemodynamic derangement, and the patient is asymptomatic. An ECG will be normal. A chest X-ray will also be normal. A large defect producing a shunt with haemodynamic significance may cause signs of heart failure, with cardiomegaly, a diastolic murmur at the apex due to increased blood flow into the left ventricle from pulmonary veins in diastole, and a loud second heart sound due to an increase in pulmonary blood flow. The ECG may show a left ventricular volume overload or biventricular hypertrophy with left ventricular hypertrophy predominant if the defect is large enough. Chest X-ray may show cardiomegaly, enlarged pulmonary arteries and increased vascular markings from pulmonary oedema, again if the defect is large.

Diagnosis

- If the defect is asymptomatic and the murmur is very suggestive of a VSD, the patient is monitored clinically. 80% of the defects close spontaneously, and hence a reassuring line can be taken. Prophylactic antibiotics are indicated for surgical and dental procedures.
- If the defect is haemodynamically significant, or if there is doubt about the diagnosis, an echocardiography should be performed. If the lesion is large enough to be symptomatic, echocardiography is essential to confirm the diagnosis and assess the shunt size.

Treatment

In haemodynamically significant defects, treatment is indicated. Medical management aims to control congestive cardiac failure and prevent the development of pulmonary vascular disease, with the maintenance of normal growth using calorie supplementation if appropriate – see gastrointestinal system. This involves the use of diuretics and angiotensin converting enzyme inhibitors such as captopril.

Surgical management is reserved for those not responding to medical management with a significant shunt. The size of the intracardiac shunt is usually expressed as the ratio of pulmonary to systemic blood flow. If the cardiac shunt is small, i.e. pulmonary to systemic flow ratio less than 2:1, the cardiac chambers are unlikely to be enlarged and the pulmonary bed is likely to be normal. If the shunt is large with a pulmonary to systemic flow ratio greater then 2:1, left atrial and ventricular volume overload occur and there is significantly raised pulmonary arterial pressure leading to pulmonary hypertension. This will ultimately lead to irreversible damage and the development of Eisenmenger's syndrome (see later). Cardiac surgery is usually considered if the pulmonary to systemic flow ratio is greater than 2:1. This is usually done towards the end of the first year. In complicated cases with pulmonary hypertension that are not suitable for early surgery, pulmonary artery banding is sometimes carried out e.g. multiple VSDs – 'Swiss cheese' defect.

ATRIAL SEPTAL DEFECT

This is a very common short case.

INSTRUCTION
Examine this child's heart

This is a different request to 'examine this child's cardiovascular system'. The examiners may require you to move straight to the chest and begin with palpation for the apex beat etc. If in doubt as to the question asked, however, it is always best to start from the beginning – the examiners will always stop you and ask you to move on specifically to the heart if that is what they want. You are entitled to clear instructions.

PALPATION
- Apex beat normal, left parasternal heave, no thrills

AUSCULTATION
- Heart sounds both heard
- Second heart sound is widely split, with fixed splitting
- Ejection systolic murmur left sternal edge (can be no murmur). The ejection systolic murmur is due to increased flow across the right ventricular outflow tract.
- May be diastolic murmur due to high flow across the tricuspid valve, an excellent diagnostic sign.

Supplementary questions frequently asked
- How would you confirm the diagnosis?
- How would you manage the patient?
- What are the indications for surgery?

NOTES ON ATRIAL SEPTAL DEFECT

The most common site of the defect is in the fossa ovalis (ostium secundum). Other sites include the septum primum (ostium primum defect, more recently called partial AVSD) and the atrioventricular septum (atrioventricular septal defect, atrioventricular canal defect, more recently called complete AVSD). The main haemodynamic abnormality is right ventricular volume overload during diastole with an increased pulmonary blood flow secondary to the shunt. Most children are asymptomatic and the lesion is discovered on routine examination. Symptoms of an ASD rarely develop before the third decade. Patients may then go on to develop atrial arrhythmias, pulmonary hypertension and heart failure.

Investigations

- ECG
- Echocardiogram

Ostium secundum – right axis deviation, partial right bundle branch block.
Ostium primum – left axis deviation, partial right bundle branch block.

Treatment is usually surgical closure in the fourth or fifth year of life, a newer technique being developed is transcatheter closure with a device. If left untreated, the defect will cause symptoms in adult years. The procedure is considered to be low risk. Antibiotic prophylaxis required for surgical and dental procedures.

PULMONARY STENOSIS

INSTRUCTION

Listen to this child's heart

AUSCULTATION

- Ejection systolic murmur maximal at the upper left sternal edge, radiation through to the back
- Heart sounds both heard
- Ejection click
- Split second heart sound, with softer pulmonary component, even absent if stenosis is severe

FURTHER EXAMINATION

Usually normal but look for the stigmata of Noonan's syndrome or Williams' syndrome.

NOTES ON PULMONARY STENOSIS

- Haemodynamically, pulmonary stenosis causes pressure overload of the right ventricle and a relatively fixed cardiac output
- Patients are usually asymptomatic if the stenosis is mild or moderate
- Neonates can get critical pulmonary stenosis with cyanosis due to shunting across the foramen ovale. This is a separate entity and requires urgent surgery.

Investigations

- ECG – usually normal, with severe stenosis there may be evidence of right ventricular overload with RV hypertrophy and tall spiked P waves
- CXR – usually normal, although may see a prominent pulmonary artery due to post stenotic dilatation. May see prominent RA and RV
- Echocardiography – diagnostic

Surgery is usually not indicated unless there is fixed sub-valvular stenosis or grossly thickened pulmonary valves, commonly seen in Noonan's syndrome. Prognosis is excellent.

Remember, in the exam children are often seen post repair

Post repair the child is likely to have a residual systolic and diastolic murmur (secondary to pulmonary incompetence). There may be a midline sternotomy following complete repair. Younger children are likely to have had a balloon angioplasty at cardiac catheterisation which does not require open heart surgery i.e. there will be no scars.

AORTIC STENOSIS

INSTRUCTION

Examine this child's cardiovascular system

INSPECTION

- Normal

Hands

- Normal

Pulse

- May be collapsing, although usually normal. If defect severe, pulse pressure may be low causing weak peripheral pulses

Blood pressure

- Normal or slightly raised, narrow pulse pressure

PALPATION

- Supra-sternal and carotid thrill
- Apex beat may be displaced and forceful

AUSCULTATION

- Heart sounds normal
- Ejection click heard best at the lower left sternal edge and apex
- Systolic murmur at the lower left sternal edge, in the aortic area and radiating into the neck

FURTHER EXAMINATION

- Ask to feel femoral pulses and feel for radio-femoral delay as sometimes aortic stenosis is associated with coarctation
- Listen at the back to confirm (aortic stenosis does not radiate to the back – coarctation does)
- May hear the diastolic murmur of aortic incompetence, particularly post surgery (associated with this is collapsing pulse)
- In severe stenosis the second heart sound may be reduced in intensity or absent

Associations of aortic stenosis

- Turner's syndrome
- Williams' syndrome – supra-valvular aortic stenosis
- Coarctation of the aorta
- Other cardiac abnormalities e.g. hypoplastic left ventricle, mitral valve abnormalities

NOTES ON AORTIC STENOSIS

In congenital aortic stenosis the valves are abnormal with one or two cusps (bicuspid) rather than the usual three (tricuspid). The main haemodynamic effect is systolic overload (pressure overload) of the left ventricle and a fixed cardiac output. This constant pressure load stimulates left ventricular hypertrophy. Symptoms include chest pain on exertion and syncope, although most patients are asymptomatic. Syncope is important as it indicates severe disease.

Investigations

ECG is normal in mild obstruction. In severe lesions there may be left ventricular hypertrophy on the ECG, but it is often surprisingly normal. In very severe lesions there may be evidence of ischaemia.

ECG signs of left ventricular hypertrophy

- Sinus rhythm with normal axis
- Tall R waves V5 – V6
- Inverted T waves in 1, aVL, V5 – V6

ECG signs of ischaemia

- ST depression
- T wave inversion

CXR may show a prominent left ventricle.

Echocardiography is always indicated. It is diagnostic and will assess the gradient across the stenosis.

Treatment

Treatment is conservative in most cases avoiding valve replacement in the young patient. If the gradient across the valve is greater than 60 mmHg, treatment is indicated. This is usually in the form of a balloon valvuloplasty at cardiac catheter, or surgical valvuloplasty.

As with pulmonary stenosis, the patient may present post repair, with the murmur of aortic stenosis still present and the murmur of aortic regurgitation due to the residual incompetence of the valve post operatively. If the patient is older, they may have had the stenosis repaired via an open valvuloplasty and could have a median sternotomy scar. Younger children may have had a catheter repair and will not therefore have a sternotomy scar.

Supravalvular aortic stenosis

This is a diffuse/localised narrowing immediately above the aortic sinuses and the coronary arteries. Most commonly occurs as part of Williams' syndrome. Many patients have peripheral pulmonary artery stenosis in addition. Clinical presentation is similar to aortic stenosis.

Williams' syndrome

- Round facies with full cheeks and lips
- Stellate pattern in the iris
- Strabismus
- Supravalvular aortic stenosis
- Branch pulmonary artery stenosis
- Hypercalcaemia
- Mental retardation, friendly personality

Subaortic stenosis

This is a fibrous diaphragm just below the aortic valve, often associated with an abnormal sub-aortic region. It is often seen with coarctation. Clinical presentation is similar to aortic stenosis although is often not severe. There is no ejection click. Treatment consists of excision of the diaphragm in all but the mildest of cases as it can be easily performed without interfering with other structures. Sub-aortic stenosis patients are particularly prone to bacterial endocarditis.

COARCTATION OF THE AORTA

INSTRUCTION

Examine this child's cardiovascular system

INSPECTION

- Normal

Hands

- Normal

Pulses

- Right radial pulse normal
- Compare radial pulses; left radial may be absent
- Femoral pulses may be weak
- May be radio-femoral delay

Face

- Look for dysmorphic features (Turner's syndrome)

Scars

- None unless there has been a repair

NB It is likely if you see a case in the exam it will be post repair (left thoracotomy scar)

PALPATION

- Apex beat normally placed, no heaves or thrills

AUSCULTATION

- Systolic murmur – loudest at the back. Alternatively the murmur may be non-specific or absent. Ejection click at upper left sternal edge if there is a bicuspid aortic valve. There may be a diastolic murmur from collaterals in the older patient.

Supplementary questions

- Associations   Turner's syndrome
                        Bicuspid aortic valve 70%
- Over half of the patients with coarctation have other lesions e.g. VSD, mitral valve abnormalities and aortic stenosis.

NOTES ON COARCTATION OF THE AORTA

98% originate just below the origin of the left subclavian artery, at the origin of the ductus arteriosus – the juxtaductal coarctation. The remaining ones are pre-ductal and often associated with arch hypoplasia. Male:female 2:1. Pre-ductal are more serious and often present in the neonatal period due to its severity. The juxtaductal type may be mild and often do not present until late childhood. Even then they are often asymptomatic and brought to attention during the investigation of hypertension.

The classical signs are of a disparity in pulses and blood pressure between the arms and the legs, hence the pulses in the arms and legs should always be palpated together at some point in a cardiovascular examination. The delay occurs due to the fact that the blood flow to the descending aorta is dependent on collaterals, hence the femoral pulse is felt after the radial. The blood pressure difference should be measured in all four limbs. Normally, the systolic pressure in the legs is 10–20 mmHg higher than in the arms, in coarctation it is lower. If the BP is higher in the right arm than in the left, it suggests involvement of the left subclavian artery in the coarctation.

Investigation

CXR – usually normal in the juxtaductal coarctation unless it does not present until after the first decade when there may be mild to moderate cardiac enlargement due to left ventricular prominence. Rib notching occurs in children with long standing coarctation (>7 years).

ECG – usually normal unless late presentation as above, when may be signs of left ventricular hypertrophy.

Echocardiography – demonstrates the presence and position of the coarctation. Will also determine the pressure gradient across the coarctation and exclude an intracardiac abnormality.

Surgical treatment

A subclavian flap or Gore-tex graft is used to repair the abnormal segment. Repair is through a left-sided thoracotomy. Complications include residual hypertension and re-coarctation. The latter can be treated with balloon dilatation, although occasionally further surgery is required. Subclavian flap repair causes the loss of the pulse in the left arm. This could be confused with a modified Blalock-Taussig shunt, which is also performed through a thoracotomy and sometimes causes loss of the pulse. If these two signs are present, you must listen for a shunt murmur, and if it is absent and the child is not cyanosed, think of a coarctation repair with a subclavian flap.

DEXTROCARDIA

It is essential not to miss dextrocardia in the exam. Cases are quite common and readily available to the examining centre to put into the exam to catch people out. If you have any difficulty locating the apex either on palpation or auscultation it is worth checking the right side of the chest. It is probably sensible to include it in your examination as a matter of routine in order to show to the examiner that you remember to look.

Dextrocardia is when the heart apex points to the right. The term dextrocardia in association with situs inversus indicates that the left atrium is on the right, the right atrium on the left, the three lobed right lung is on the left, the two lobed left lung is on the right, the stomach and spleen are on the right and the liver is on the left. This, in association with normally related great arteries is most often a functionally normal heart. Dextrocardia without situs inversus (and levocardia with situs inversus) are most often complicated by severe cardiac malformations that include various combinations of single ventricle, arterial transposition, pulmonary stenosis, ASDs, VSDs, AVSDs, TAPVD, tricuspid atresia and pulmonary artery hypoplasia/atresia.

Abnormalities of the position of the heart are also associated with the asplenia and polysplenia syndromes.

Dextrocardia is also associated with immotile cilia syndrome, or the Kartagener's syndrome (dextrocardia, bronchiectasis, situs inversus, infertility, sinusitis, dysplasia of the frontal sinuses and otitis media).
If you find dextrocardia on examination, it is therefore important that you go on to palpate the abdomen to find the position of the liver and to listen to the lung fields for bronchiectasis.

THE CYANOSED CHILD

Cases in the exam are often quite difficult. Many will have had surgery and the cardiac lesions are likely to be complex. It is important to describe what you see and to make sensible statements about potential causes. It is therefore essential to have a good overview of cyanotic congenital heart disease. Some useful information is summarised below.

While thinking about this it is important to remember that children who have had definitive surgery for cyanotic congenital heart disease when seen in the exam will be pink e.g. transposition of the great arteries or tetralogy of Fallot and will present as a pink child with a central sternotomy scar with in some cases an additional shunt scar. Children seen in the exam who have cyanosis due to cardiac causes are likely to have complex cyanotic congenital heart disease.

Cardiac causes of cyanosis

- Decreased pulmonary blood flow e.g. tetralogy of Fallot, pulmonary atresia, Ebstein's anomaly, tricuspid atresia
- Poor mixing e.g. transposition of great arteries
- Common mixing e.g. truncus arteriosus, double outlet right ventricle, total anomalous pulmonary venous drainage, univentricular heart

Management

Fallot's tetralogy – see page 35

Pulmonary atresia with or without an intact intra-ventricular septum, difficult problem usually requires several shunt procedures, definitive repair often not possible.

Transposition of the great arteries is the second commonest cyanotic lesion, comprising 4% of all congenital disease. Infants at presentation need a prostaglandin infusion, followed by urgent transfer to a cardiology unit. Treatment has recently changed. Until approximately 5 years ago, a balloon atrial septostomy was performed, the infant returned home to thrive and then a permanent procedure was carried out at 6–9 months (Mustard or Senning operations). Now, in some centres, the arterial duct is maintained by a prostaglandin infusion and a definitive repair is carried out within the first few days (arterial switch).

Truncus arteriosus, rare comprising 0.5% of all lesions. Often associated with chromosomal abnormality (22q deletion syndrome).

Double outlet right ventricle, rare. Early pulmonary banding or shunt procedure followed by definitive repair at a later date.

Total anomalous pulmonary venous drainage, rare, comprising 1% of all cardiac cases (40% have other associated cardiac lesions). Definitive repair early.

Univentricular heart – as common as transposition, in certain series published, 4%. Many different types. No correction only palliation. Often die early. If cyanosis severe may need shunt procedure early. Pulmonary artery banding if the pulmonary artery pressure high, new shunts as the patient grows. If reach 5 years, surgery to palliate the defect involving Fontan/modified Fontan procedure – total cavo-pulmonary anastomoses, bypass the right side of the heart.

CASE SCENARIOS

The following are examples of cases of cyanotic heart disease we have seen within our hospital, which are the classical types and typical of cases seen in the exam.

Case 1

8-month-old girl. She appears small for her age although I would like to plot her on a centile chart. She is tachypnoeic at rest. She is centrally cyanosed. She has no dysmorphic features. She is clubbed and has peripheral cyanosis. She has an absent right brachial and radial pulse, there is no radio-femoral delay. She has a right sided thoracotomy scar. On auscultation she has a normal first heart sound and a single second heart sound. She has a continuous murmur over the right side of her chest. (At the end of this examination you should suggest palpating the abdomen for a liver and taking the blood pressure.)

This set of clinical signs would fit with a child with a complex cyanotic congenital heart lesion who has had a shunt procedure.

Possible diagnoses include
- pulmonary atresia without a VSD
- double outlet right ventricle
- univentricular heart with pulmonary atresia

Notes

You would not be expected to come up with that diagnosis, but carefully eliciting the clinical signs will allow a best guess. In this case, with the shunt and the single second heart sound, a diagnosis of pulmonary atresia would be the first best guess. Fallot's is less likely because there is no systolic murmur of pulmonary stenosis and in pulmonary stenosis there should be 2 components of the second sound.

Case 2

20-month-old girl. She appears to be thriving although I would like to plot her on a centile chart. She has no dysmorphic features and appears to be comfortable at rest. She is mildly cyanosed centrally. Her pulses are normal throughout. She has no radiofemoral delay. She has a median sternotomy scar but no thoracotomy scars. Her apex beat is localised to the 5th intercostal space on the right, there are no heaves or thrills. She has normal heart sounds on the right side and appears to have dextrocardia. There is continuous murmur

---

This set of clinical signs would fit with a child with a complex congenital cardiac defect who is likely to have had a central shunt procedure e.g. cavopulmonary anastomoses. These are performed in children in whom definitive repair of their cardiac defect is not possible and effectively bypass the right side of the heart. The case described had a complex cardiac defect involving right atrial isomerism, dextrocardia, a complete AV canal defect and a single ventricle with pulmonary atresia. Again, as in the case above, a precise diagnosis would not be expected.

Notes

If the heart sounds are difficult to hear, as a matter of routine listen to the right side of the chest to exclude dextrocardia. Mild cyanosis in a child with a median sternotomy scar suggests a palliative shunt procedure for those children in whom definitive surgery is not possible.

Case 3

13-year-old girl. She has facial features of Down's syndrome. She is deeply cyanosed at rest. She is clubbed and peripherally cyanosed. Her pulses are normal in character and the rate is... There is no radio femoral delay. There are no scars visible on the thorax. Her apex beat is... On auscultation she has a normal first heart sound, a loud second heart sound and a pansystolic murmur, maximal at the left sternal edge but heard all over the chest. I would like to go on and palpate her abdomen for a liver.

This young girl with Down's syndrome is most likely to have AVSD with shunt reversal resulting in Eisenmenger's syndrome. This was the diagnosis in this girl.

Notes

Down's syndrome children who have no scars and are cyanosed at the age of thirteen are likely to have a defect causing Eisenmenger's – be prepared to talk about Eisenmenger's syndrome and its prognosis. This case could just as well be a long case in view of the issue of Down's syndrome and cardiac surgery and, specifically in our case, the complicating factor of parents who are Jehovah's witnesses – a very good long case!

Eisenmenger's syndrome

Children with Down's syndrome are at particular risk of developing Eisenmenger's syndrome. This is a condition in which there is pulmonary hypertension due to high pulmonary vascular resistance, with a reversed or bi-directional shunt at aortopulmonary, ventricular or atrial level. It may occur in patent ductus arteriosus, aortopulmonary window, ventricular septal defect or atrial septal defect. It has also been applied to more complex defects when a very high pulmonary vascular resistance causes a dominant right to left shunt, such as persistent truncus, single ventricle, single atrium, atrioventricular defect and total anomalous pulmonary venous drainage. When Eisenmenger's occurs the defect must be large, although children with Down's syndrome and ventricular septal defect or atrioventricular septal defect are particularly liable to develop pulmonary hypertension and reversal of shunt at an early age. It occurs much later in patent ductus arteriosus and atrial septal defect.

Patients are generally cyanosed with clubbing and signs are those of pulmonary hypertension. The pulse is of normal volume. There is a right ventricular heave. There is a short ejection systolic murmur (ejection of blood into the dilated pulmonary artery) often preceded by an ejection click and a very loud second heart sound. The chest X-ray shows right ventricular prominence with small peripheral pulmonary vessels. The ECG shows peaked 'P' waves due to right atrial hypertrophy, right axis deviation and moderate or marked right ventricular hypertrophy with tall R waves in V4R and V1.

Treatment is difficult, surgical closure is not possible and there is no known medical treatment that will influence pulmonary vascular resistance. Heart-lung transplant is the only life saving procedure.

FALLOT'S TETRALOGY

This is a classic short case and frequently seen. It will usually have been operated on by the time the child is seen.

TYPICAL CASE

Age 6 months

INSPECTION

- Cyanosed
- Failure to thrive

Hands

- Early clubbing

Pulse

- Normal
- May be absent left sided pulse in association with left thoracotomy scar (or a similar situation on the right) – see below

Blood pressure

- Normal

Face

- Central cyanosis

Scars

- If untreated, none
- May be left/right thoracotomy scar in association with an absent pulse on the corresponding side (classical Blalock-Taussig shunt – usually right side performed first, modified Blalock-Taussig shunt – Gore-tex conduit side to side from the subclavian artery to the homolateral branch of the pulmonary artery). There may be bilateral thoracotomy scars suggesting the failure of one shunt and the need for a second shunt procedure (not uncommon). There may be a central sternotomy scar which indicates definitive repair has been carried out. If the definitive repair has been carried out the child will not be cyanosed.

PALPATION

- Apex beat normally located sub-sternal
- Right ventricular impulse
- 50% have a systolic thrill palpable at the left sternal edge

AUSCULTATION

Murmurs

- Loud systolic murmur maximal at left sternal edge, transmitted widely especially to the lungs. May be ejection systolic or pansystolic and is caused by turbulence across the right ventricular outflow tract.
- Shunt murmur

Heart sounds

- The second heart sound is either single or the pulmonary component is soft

NOTES ON FALLOT'S TETRALOGY

The constituents of Fallot's tetralogy are

- obstruction to right ventricular outflow tract
- VSD
- overriding aorta
- right ventricular hypertrophy

Investigations

Hb/PCV – if cyanosed
CXR – prominent right ventricle, small pulmonary arteries, pulmonary oligaemia
ECG – right axis deviation, right ventricular hypertrophy. P wave is tall and peaked.
Echo – demonstrates the lesion and the size of the pulmonary arteries and side of aorta, obviating the need for cardiac catheterisation

Treatment

Depends on the severity of the right ventricular outflow tract obstruction. If it is severe then a palliative shunt procedure may be performed as above. This decreases the amount of hypoxia and allows increases in linear growth as well as growth of the main pulmonary arteries. Corrective surgery can then take place. The optimum time for corrective surgery varies from child to child and depends on the clinical severity of the lesion, the type of anatomy demonstrated at investigation and the size of the child. There is a wide spectrum of severity and it depends on individual cardiology review. The current recommendation is that surgery is carried out between 6 and 12 months of age.

Complications

- Exertional dyspnoea – squat for relief
- Paroxysmal hypercyanotic spells
- Cerebral thrombosis/brain abscess

Paroxysmal hypercyanotic spells

The infant becomes restless and cyanotic, with increasing cyanosis, gasping respiration may occur followed by syncope. The attacks are most common after exertion and during the first two years of life.

Treatment

1. Bring baby's knees to chest (reduces venous return and increases systemic resistance, reversing the shunt)
2. Morphine
3. Sodium bicarbonate if acidotic
4. Vasoconstrictors
5. Beta blockers

COMPLEX CONGENITAL HEART DISEASE – POST REPAIR

Many of the cardiac cases seen in the exam will have had surgery, often definitive. In some cases it is clear what surgery has been carried out and the underlying diagnosis is clear. For example, a child who is pink with an absent left brachial pulse and a left lateral thoracotomy scar has probably had a coarctation repair. In other cases it is less clear, such as the child with a central sternotomy scar who may have had straightforward surgery, e.g. VSD or the repair of complicated congenital heart disease. We have tried to illustrate this in the cases described above and would advise candidates that if such cases are seen and are not straightforward, discussion should be in the most general terms only.

Case

This is a 3-year-old boy. He looks well and is not tachypnoeic at rest. His right radial pulse is absent. He has a scar from cardiac catheterisation. He has a right thoracotomy scar and midline sternotomy scar. I presume he has complex congenital heart disease, now repaired, and I would like to proceed to listen to the heart...

It is not possible to achieve a specific diagnosis in this case.

YOUR NOTES

YOUR NOTES

CHAPTER 2 – RESPIRATORY MEDICINE

The respiratory examination is straightforward and should be revised thoroughly and practised frequently. The conditions seen are common – cystic fibrosis, other chronic suppurative lung disease, asthma and bronchopulmonary dysplasia. Studying these conditions well will present a good opportunity for you to score highly if you see them in the exam.

SUMMARY

- Scheme for examination of the respiratory system
- Signs of respiratory distress
- Causes of clubbing
- Hyperexpansion
- Harrison's sulcus
- Lateral thoracotomy scars
- Asthma
- Bronchiolitis
- Cystic fibrosis
- Bronchiectasis
- Primary ciliary dyskinesia
- Bronchopulmonary dysplasia
- Kyphoscoliosis
- Stridor
- Causes of an enlarged tongue
- Tracheostomy

SCHEME FOR EXAMINATION OF THE RESPIRATORY SYSTEM

Find your own system with which you are comfortable. It is important to start with a general assessment looking for dysmorphology, nutritional status and any other specific features. The following is a suggested scheme.

Baby

It is reasonable to change the order of examination to gain the maximum information before the baby starts to cry. You need to develop your own scheme to include the following:

- Observation – dysmorphology, thriving, cyanosis, recession, respiratory rate, chest expansion, scars
- Auscultation
- Percussion
- Clubbing
- Anaemia
- Trachea position
- Apex beat and heart sounds
- Hepatomegaly
- ENT

Older child

- Look from end of bed for wasting, inhalers/nebulizers, pancreatic enzymes, peak flow meter, sputum pot, BCG scar
- Assess chest expansion
- Examine for pectus excavatum and Harrison's sulci
- Examine hands for clubbing, cyanosis and anaemia
- Count pulse and respiratory rate
- Assess respiratory effort (nasal flaring, recession, tracheal tug)
- Look in the mouth for central cyanosis
- Feel suprasternal notch for tracheal deviation
- Lift each arm in turn and look for scars (e.g. lateral thoracotomy)
- Palpate apex beat (mediastinal shift)
- Percuss (anteriorly, posteriorly and laterally)
- Auscultate (anteriorly, posteriorly and laterally)

At the end of your examination

- Ask to examine the ears, nose and throat, see sputum specimen and perform peak flow measurement (if appropriate)
- Assess for tactile vocal fremitus, vocal resonance if appropriate (e.g. suspected consolidation)

Different instructions may be given and you need to adapt your examination accordingly

- Examine this child's chest
- Examine this child's respiratory system
- Look at this child's chest and tell me what you see – hyper-expansion, thoracotomy scars, Harrison's sulci, wasting
- Just listen to this child's chest
- Perform a peak flow measurement on this child
- The GP says this child does not have asthma – do you agree? – the examiner is expecting you to comment on the child's hyper-expansion.

NOTES ON EXAMINATION OF THE RESPIRATORY SYSTEM

Signs of respiratory distress

- Audible wheeze
- Tachypnoea
- Tachycardia
- Nasal flaring
- Intercostal/subcostal/sternal/supra-sternal recession
- Drowsiness and confusion
- Cyanosis

Causes of clubbing

- Bronchiectasis/cystic fibrosis
- Primary ciliary dyskinesia
- Pulmonary tuberculosis
- Fibrosing alveolitis
- Empyema/lung abscess
- Malignancy
- Cyanotic congenital heart disease
- Bacterial endocarditis
- Biliary cirrhosis
- Chronic active hepatitis
- Inflammatory bowel disease

How to assess clubbing

This can be difficult if early but is often asked. The first changes of clubbing are loss of the nail fold angle (most easily seen by asking the child to hold the thumbs together nail to nail and looking through the gap) and a fluctuant bogginess of the nail bed. Increased curvature of the nail bed and enlargement of the distal phalanx occur later.

Hyperexpansion

This implies chest disease and is an extremely important physical sign. Practise the assessment of hyperexpansion. Look from the front first and then assess by looking at the child from the side and examining antero-posterior diameter and its excursion during the respiratory phases. Comment on asymmetry if seen.

Causes of hyperexpansion – common conditions seen in the exam

- Asthma
- Cystic fibrosis
- Bronchiectasis – see below for list of causes

- Bronchopulmonary dysplasia – look for neonatal sequelae e.g. head shape, chest drain/IV scars

Others

- Recurrent aspiration

- Repaired tracheo-oesophageal fistula

Harrison's sulcus

Harrison's sulcus is visible as a bilateral fixed indrawing of the anterior portion of the lower ribs. It is caused by chronic airway obstruction encouraging excessive diaphragmatic use which causes deformity where the diaphragm inserts into the ribcage. Its presence therefore suggests long-standing airway obstruction.

**Hyperexpanded chest *plus* clubbing implies
cystic fibrosis or bronchiectasis**

**Hyperexpanded chest *without* clubbing implies
asthma or bronchopulmonary dysplasia**

ASTHMA

Children with asthma are commonly brought down from the ward to cover a shortfall in cases.

INSTRUCTION

Examine this child's chest
Comment on the appearance of this child's chest
Check this child's peak flow
Asthma – in patient ready for discharge – summarise your assessment

---

Case

Simon is a well looking caucasian boy who appears well grown for his age. There is no clubbing or cyanosis. On inspection of his chest he has bilateral Harrison's sulci. His respiratory rate is 48 bpm. Auscultation of his chest reveals bilateral expiratory wheeze with a prolonged expiratory component. The most likely diagnosis is asthma. I would also like to ask Simon to perform a peak flow measurement...

Clinical examination

General appearance –
- Hyperexpansion, chest wall deformity – Harrison's sulci, pectus carinatum
- Signs of respiratory distress
- Wheeze and prolonged expiration
- Peak flow

also look for
clubbing, wasting, coarse crepitations, focal signs, central lines, neonatal scars – all make alternative diagnosis more likely

NB Clubbing is not seen in children with just asthma.

Differential diagnoses of asthma – you may be asked this

- Causes of bronchiectasis (see later)
- Bronchiolitis (infants)
- Bronchopulmonary dysplasia
- Congestive cardiac failure (myocarditis/CHD)
- H-type tracheo-oesophageal fistula
- Tracheo-oesophageal fistula – post repair
- Vascular ring
- Gastro-oesophageal reflux
- Lymphadenopathy (TB/Hodgkin's/sarcoidosis)

NOTES ON ASTHMA

Epidemiology

Prevalence 10% of pre-school rising to 30% of school age children. Three-fold increase in past 40 years. 1% of asthmatic children admitted to hospital each year. 50 deaths per year under age 16 in the UK.

Management

The aim is to achieve normal activity and use inhaled bronchodilators less than twice per week.

General measures

These include damp dusting, washing toys, avoiding cigarette smoke and animal dander.

Drug therapy

Acute attacks are treated with inhaled or nebulised beta 2 agonists and oral steroids. More severe acute attacks are managed with intravenous aminophylline, salbutamol and hydrocortisone, and occasionally ventilation. Long-term treatment is with inhaled prophylactic steroids. The device selected for drug delivery is important and age specific. It is necessary to be familiar with all the inhaler and spacer devices and the most appropriate age at which to use them. Familiarise yourself also with the latest British Thoracic Society guidelines for the treatment of chronic asthma in children.

Delivery devices

You will need to be able to discuss these in some detail and be able to demonstrate their use to the examiner. Many candidates who attend Part Two clinical courses are unable to use many of the devices correctly. This does not give the examiner a good impression.

For babies and toddlers, up to the age of 5 years, the most efficient delivery system is a metered dose inhaler coupled to a spacer device (e.g. volumatic/nebuhaler). The spacer slows down the particles and requires no co-ordination to use. For under twos who are unable to breathe directly into the mouthpiece a soft rubber mask is supplied. Spacers must be replaced when they become scratched and when they are cleaned they must be left to drip-dry, and not wiped with a cloth as the static charge produced reduces the availability of the particles. Most toddlers cope well with this device. Babies tolerate it less well, it may be worth changing to a device with a smaller volume and a more pliant valve to match the tidal volume of the baby (e.g. *Babyhaler*). If this does not work then it may be necessary to deliver the medication via a home nebuliser.

At age 5 years there is a wide choice of inhaler devices. Dry powder inhalers such as the diskhaler can be very useful and are easy to carry to school. You will need to learn the technique of loading and using this inhaler as it is different from all the others. *Turbohalers* are simpler to use and are popular with school children; the *Accuhaler which is* another dry powder inhaler is said to be one of the easiest to use. *Easibreathe* and *Autohaler* devices are self activating with a propellant, the child still needs to be able to take a deep breath and hold it when using them.

Chloro-fluoro-carbon free inhalers are being introduced from 1999

Try to find an example of each of the different asthma devices in your hospital and get someone experienced to help you practise handling them and be able to explain to a parent (or the examiner) how they are used.

Summary of devices

- Home nebulizer
- Spacer devices   volumatic/Nebuhaler/Babyhaler + face mask
- Dry powder   Accuhaler, Diskhaler, Turbohaler, Rotahaler (used rarely)
- Self actuating with   Autohaler/Easibreathe/Clickhaler propellant
- Metered dose inhalers

You may be asked to summarise your assessment of an asthmatic child ready for discharge

Include the following points:

- Adjust the child's medication if appropriate – did under treatment precipitate the admission, is the child's bronchodilator usage high suggesting poor control and is there a need to increase prophylactic medication?
- Check patient is stable on the medication they will receive at home
- Check inhaler/spacer and peak flow technique and adjust as necessary
- Explain in basic terms the difference between bronchospasm and inflammation and the relevance of using a regular preventative steroid in that context
- Provide a written action plan with clear instructions of what to do if the asthma worsens
- Provide a peak flow diary
- Give advice on avoiding precipitants
- Write to the GP
- Arrange community or asthma nurse to visit, e.g. if there are concerns over compliance
- Arrange appropriate follow-up

Remember you must be familiar with how to use the medication prescribed and may be asked to explain it to a proxy patient

BRONCHIOLITIS

There are many stable infants with bronchiolitis in the winter and they are commonly used as short cases – particularly if there is a shortage of other cases.

Case

Jade is 6 months old. She appears to be well grown. I would like to plot her on a growth chart. She is in headbox oxygen and is in respiratory distress with tachypnoea of 80 bpm, nasal flaring and intercostal recession. There is no cyanosis. Auscultation of her chest reveals bilateral inspiratory and expiratory wheeze and bilateral fine crepitations. The most likely diagnosis is bronchiolitis...

NOTES ON BRONCHIOLITIS

Bronchiolitis is an acute viral respiratory illness affecting infants up to 1 year of age (peak incidence at 6 months). It occurs in winter epidemics. Main causative agent is respiratory syncytial virus in 50% of cases (sero-types A and B), remainder is due to parainfluenza, mycoplasma and adenovirus. Infants are more at risk of developing bronchiolitis if their parents smoke and if they live in crowded conditions. Breast feeding is partially protective, presumably through passive transfer of anti-RSV immunoglobulin. Examination reveals tachypnoea, recession, hyperexpansion, bilateral wheeze and crackles. Consolidation is found in 30% of patients and is usually due to atelectasis.

Differential diagnoses include

- Heart disease   VSD/AVSD
  myocarditis
  total anomalous pulmonary venous drainage
- Bronchopneumonia   bacterial (staphylococcal)
  aspiration
  pertussis
- Post viral wheeze
- Foreign body

High risk group

- Congenital heart disease
- Cystic fibrosis
- Bronchopulmonary dysplasia
- Immunodeficiency

Prognosis is slightly worse in the high risk group (mortality 3.5% v. 1%)

Management

Supportive, providing help with feeding (nasogastric feeds or intravenous fluids). Supplementary oxygen by headbox or nasal cannula with additional respiratory support either by continuous airway pressure or ventilation if appropriate. Frequent monitoring is clearly necessary. Suction and saline nose drops are important as secretions are usually profuse and contribute to the airway obstruction and poor feeding. Ipratropium bromide via nebulizer reverses some of the short-term effects of bronchiolitis but has not been shown to alter mortality or length of stay in hospital. More recently there has been considerable interest in the use of nebulised adrenaline.

Ribavirin is normally reserved for the sickest infants. It reduces viral shedding and shortens the duration of illness but has not been shown to cause a reduction in mortality. Steroids are of some use in obliterative bronchiolitis, a destructive form of bronchiolitis, usually associated with adenovirus and resulting in bronchiectasis.

CYSTIC FIBROSIS

Cystic fibrosis patients are seen very commonly in the exam. A thorough knowledge of all aspects of this condition is required.

INSTRUCTION

Examine this child's chest – crackles/wheeze/central line
Examine this child's hands – clubbing
Look at this child – wasting/nasogastric tube
Examine this child's abdomen – gastrostomy/scars/ hepatosplenomegaly
Examine this child's chest – what else would you like to examine – abdomen, nutritional status, ENT, cardiac

General examination

- Height and weight
- Cyanosis, supplemental oxygen
- Visible central line or gastrostomy
- Obvious hyperexpansion and respiratory distress
- Scars – thoracotomy, abdominal
- Wasting – muscle bulk (mid-arm circumference), subcutaneous fat (skin fold thickness)
- Pancreatic enzymes, peak flow and nebulizers in evidence

Case – 15-year-old boy

John is lying in bed, comfortable at rest. There is a central line and gastrostomy tube in situ. He looks thin with a poor muscle bulk and reduced subcutaneous fat. I would like to plot him on a height and weight chart. He is obviously hyperexpanded and using his accessory muscles of respiration. I would like to count his respiratory rate. Looking at his hands he appears clubbed...

Hands/face

- Clubbing – in older child; CF unlikely in the absence of clubbing
- Peripheral and central cyanosis
- Pulse
- Pallor
- Jaundice

Chest

- Tachypnoea
- Hyperexpansion
- Crepitations, wheeze
- Peak flow
- Sputum sample

Abdomen

- Scars – meconium ileus
- Gastrostomy
- Caput medusae
- Ascites
- Hepatosplenomegaly
- Rectal prolapse
- Palpable faeces-meconium ileus equivalent

ENT

- Nasal polyps

Others

Cardiovascular system
- Signs of right-sided heart failure secondary to pulmonary hypertension (raised JVP, dependent oedema, hepatomegaly)

Endocrine
- Growth and pubertal status

Joints
- Arthritis – occasional

NOTES ON CLINICAL FEATURES OF CYSTIC FIBROSIS

- Nutritional status is one of the most important factors in assessing a patient with cystic fibrosis. They should have their height and weight plotted on centile charts every three months; if there is concern triceps and subscapular skinfold thickness can be measured with calipers and compared to normal values.
- Meconium ileus is the presenting feature for 15% of patients.
- Meconium ileus equivalent (distal intestinal obstruction syndrome) occurs in older children (20%) presenting as cramping abdominal

pains and a palpable mass in the right iliac fossa. Treatment is with enemas of water soluble contrast (Gastrografin) to loosen the impaction.

- Rectal prolapse occurs in up to 20% (toddler presentation) and is caused by a combination of steatorrhoea and coughing. It usually resolves on starting pancreatic replacement therapy.
- Patients may present in the neonatal period with obstructive jaundice due to inspissated bile. Older children can develop focal biliary cirrhosis and 2% of these progress to multilobular cirrhosis with portal hypertension and oesophageal varices.
- Cor pulmonale can develop in the second decade secondary to severe lung disease; it is recognised by a raised jugular venous pressure, hepatomegaly and oedema. Mean survival subsequently is eight months.
- Insulin dependent diabetes occurs in 7% of patients, secondary to pancreatic fibrosis. It is easily controlled and diabetic ketoacidosis is rare, however as patients survive longer evidence of microangiopathy is now emerging.
- Arthritis occurs in 1% and seems to improve with lung function.

BACKGROUND INFORMATION ON CYSTIC FIBROSIS

Inheritance autosomal recessive. Prevalence 1:2000, carrier frequency 1:20. CFTR is a cAMP mediated chloride channel. In the lungs, normal CFTR causes efflux of chloride ions across apical membranes of the submucosal glands. Sodium and water follow. Abnormal CFTR (reduced production, defective processing or ATP-binding site defects) cause an inability to secrete chloride, sodium and then water, resulting in viscid secretions, the hallmark of CF. A similar problem occurs in the pancreatic and biliary ducts. However in the skin the function of sweat glands is to absorb chloride from the isotonic sweat. CFTR defects therefore cause a high sweat chloride, the basis of the sweat test.

Inspissated mucus in the bronchi causes failure to clear pathogenic organisms. These then colonise the airways and the resulting inflammatory reaction predisposes to repeated infections and chronic suppurative lung disease.

Genetics

There are more than 300 alterations at the gene locus on chromosome 7, at least 230 are associated with the disease. Delta F508 is the commonest mutation and is present in 75% of patients (2/3 homozygous, 1/3 heterozygous for Delta F508 and one other mutation). Different phenotypes exist, e.g. all Delta F508 patients have pancreatic insufficiency whereas R117H have some preservation of pancreatic function.

Diagnosis

- Antenatal chorionic villous sampling (8–10/40), amniocentesis (16–18/40) for gene analysis if mutation within family has been previously identified
- Guthrie test looking at immunoreactive trypsin (some centres)
- Genetic analysis
- Sweat test

MANAGEMENT OF CYSTIC FIBROSIS

Emphasis is on multidisciplinary outpatient based management, involving medical staff, physiotherapist, dietician, community nurses, social workers and psychologist as required.

- Physiotherapy – uses vibration to loosen mucus and gravity to drain it. Ideally 20 minutes twice a day for life. Normally performed by chest percussion head down over a foam wedge. Forced expiratory technique-performing 'huffs' from medium to low lung volume aids clearance. Alternatively, the patient may use breaths through a positive expiratory pressure mask followed by coughing. A regular exercise programme is beneficial.
- Antibiotics – aim to reduce colonisation with *Staphylococcus* and *Haemophilus* in infants and *Pseudomonas* in older children. Flucloxacillin is used either prophylactically before colonisation or long-term after colonisation. Nebulised colomycin or gentamicin can be used in *Pseudomonas* colonisation and some centres advocate a two week course of IV antibiotics every three months in such individuals. Acute infections are treated as they arise. Organisms can normally be predicted or isolated and oral (ciprofloxacin) or IV (ceftazidime/gentamicin/piperacillin) therapy can be started as appropriate. Patients have altered

pharmacokinetics and so higher doses are used for longer duration.

- Nutritional status is strongly correlated with the severity of pulmonary disease. Patients with cystic fibrosis suffer because they have increased metabolic demands, malabsorption and poor appetites. Most need pancreatic enzyme supplements in pH sensitive polymer capsules. The dose is titrated against growth and steatorrhoea. High lipase concentration capsules have been shown to cause colonic strictures. Patients should consult a dietician to receive a high-calorie, high-protein diet. This can be supplemented by high-calorie drinks. Overnight naso-gastric feeds are an alternative as the appetite is often poor, and eventually patients with severe weight loss may benefit from overnight gastrostomy feeds. Vitamin A, D and E supplementation is necessary.
- Treatment of co-existent conditions such as asthma and constipation (meconium ileus equivalent)
- Treatment of complications such as liver disease
- Heart lung transplant (adults with cystic fibrosis 70% survival at 1 year, 40% at 5 years)
- Gene therapy, using vectors such as liposomes or replication-deficient adenovirus to transfer normal CFTR into host cells. Still in early stages.
- DNAase, acts to digest viscous DNA derived from inflammatory cells in bronchial exudates. Most can expect a 10% increase in FEV_1 in the first week. Expensive.
- Terminal care

BRONCHIECTASIS

The chest presentation is as for cystic fibrosis and cystic fibrosis is part of the differential diagnosis of bronchiectasis.

Aetiology

- Immunodeficiency – hypogammaglobulinaemia, IgA deficiency
- Alpha 1 antitrypsin deficiency
- Foreign body
- Lobar sequestration
- Pertussis
- Primary ciliary dyskinesia
- Bronchiolitis obliterans
- Recurrent aspiration (H-TOF)
- Asthma
- Idiopathic

Treatment

- Regular physiotherapy
- Regular spirometry
- Prophylactic antibiotics
- Regular sputum cultures to detect colonising organism and its sensitivities
- Bronchodilators as bronchospasm is usually a prominent feature
- Prompt immunisation including influenza
- Mucolytics when appropriate
- Monitor for cor pulmonale

- Monitoring growth and nutrition is very important (combination of increased metabolic rate and reduced intake). Offer nutritional supplements if necessary or feed in alternative ways e.g. overnight nasogastric or gastrostomy feeds.
- Lobectomy if necessary

PRIMARY CILIARY DYSKINESIA

This is an autosomal recessive group of disorders, the most common being Kartagener's syndrome.

Features

- Bronchiectasis
- Nasal polyps
- Sinusitis
- Chronic suppurative otitis media
- Infertility

Kartagener's syndrome
(approximately 50% of primary ciliary dyskinesia)

- Bronchiectasis
- Dextrocardia
- Visceral situs inversus
- Chronic sinusitis

Case

Peter is a well looking boy who appears small for his age and I would like to plot him on the appropriate height and weight centile charts. On examination he has clubbing, and is not cyanosed. Palpation of his apex beat reveals dextrocardia and auscultation of his chest reveals coarse crepitations at both bases. The most likely diagnosis is Kartagener's syndrome. I would like to examine the abdomen and enquire about a history of sinusitis...

NOTES ON CILIARY DYSKINESIA

The mucociliary escalator works to waft mucus from the lower airways in a cephalic direction from where it is usually swallowed. Primary ciliary dyskinesia (PCD) occurs in 1:30,000 of the population. It usually presents with bronchiectasis after a troublesome period of sinusitis, nasal polyps and chronic suppurative otitis media. The cilia look grossly normal but have ultrastructural defects of the dynein side arms. A useful initial test is to place a drop of saccharin on the nasal mucosa and measure the time until a sweet taste is sensed in the mouth (normally 11 minutes). Electron microscopy of naso-ciliary brushing will reveal ultrastructural abnormalities. Finally, motility can be assessed by photometry. Prognosis: normal lifespan if properly treated.

NOTES ON OTHER CAUSES OF BRONCHIECTASIS

Immunodeficiency

- Bruton's hypogammaglobulinaemia
- Complement deficiency
- Chronic granulomatous disease
- Hyper IgE (Job's) syndrome
- AIDS

Lobar sequestration

- Non-functioning mass of embryonic tissue within chest which receives its entire arterial supply from the aorta
- Haemoptysis common
- Continuous murmur over lesion
- Needs aortography before removal because feeding vessel usually arises from abdomen

BRONCHOPULMONARY DYSPLASIA (BPD)/CHRONIC LUNG DISEASE OF INFANCY

This is a very common short case

Cases – 6-month-old boy

Jordan looks small for his age. I would like to plot his weight, length and head circumference on a centile chart. There is no clubbing. He has a hyperexpanded chest. There is mild intercostal recession. He has two chest drain scars on the right and the dorsum of both hands have venepuncture scars. Auscultation of the chest reveals bilateral wheeze. The most likely diagnosis is bronchopulmonary dysplasia.

I would like to perform a developmental examination...

NB May be oxygen dependent so look out for oxygen tubing and oxygen cylinder.

NOTES ON BRONCHOPULMONARY DYSPLASIA (BPD)

The definition of bronchopulmonary dysplasia states that the child must have been ventilated after birth and be oxygen dependent at 28 days with evidence of lung disease or an abnormal chest X-ray. The prevalence is 20% of all ventilated babies rising to 70% of babies ventilated for more than two weeks.

Associations: ventilated with a peak pressure greater than 35 cmH_2O, prematurity, patent ductus arteriosus, air leak.

Presentation in the exam will be an infant who is obviously small for its age. Note that the head may have a characteristic scaphocephalic appearance and the face may look cushingoid (dexamethasone). The best visual clues are chest drain or venesection scars. Comment on the presence of cyanosis (unlikely in the exam), or respiratory distress. There may be stridor (prolonged intubation) or wheeze and the chest is usually hyperexpanded. A thoracotomy scar suggests patent ductus arteriosus ligation. Ask to examine the heart, in particular, for a patent ductus, or a loud second heart sound of pulmonary hypertension. There may be an abdominal scar for a Nissen's fundoplication or gastrostomy. Always consider a developmental examination.

Differential diagnoses of this picture

- Other causes of hyperexpanded chest/bronchiectasis – see earlier
- Immunodeficiency e.g. severe combined immunodeficiency/chronic granulomatous disease
- Chronic aspiration (gastro-oesophageal reflux/repaired tracheo-oesophageal fistula)
- Congenital heart disease (e.g. AVSD), cardiac failure

Treatment

- Supplemental oxygen to maintain good saturations
- Dexamethasone if necessary – particularly to aid weaning off the ventilator
- Physiotherapy as appropriate
- Nutrition – additional calories are frequently required
- Assess for complications e.g. patent ductus, right-sided heart failure
- Gastro-oesophageal reflux is frequently present and a trial of therapy is worthwhile in difficult cases

KYPHOSCOLIOSIS

Positional if disappears on bending down, otherwise it is structural and pathological.

Causes

Commonly

- Idiopathic (usually in pre-pubertal girls)
- Cerebral palsy

Others

- Duchenne muscular dystrophy
- Poliomyelitis
- Spinal muscular atrophy (type II/III)
- Friedreich's ataxia
- Neurofibromatosis type 1
- Marfan's syndrome
- Homocystinuria
- Osteogenesis imperfecta
- Klippel-Feil sequence (fused cervical vertebrae, webbed neck, facial asymmetry, deafness, VSD, renal anomalies, Sprengel-shoulder)
- Alagille's syndrome (broad forehead, prominent chin, posterior embryotoxon-opaque border to cornea, peripheral pulmonary artery stenosis, butterfly vertebrae, cholestasis)
- Mucopolysaccharidoses (short, large head, macroglossia, hepato-splenomegaly, cloudy cornea in Hurler's)

NOTES ON KYPHOSCOLIOSIS

Scoliosis is the lateral curvature of the spine accompanied by rotation of the vertebral bodies and viscera. It causes a reduction in chest wall compliance and its major importance is reduction in lung volumes causing a restrictive defect. The earliest manifestation of this is a fall in PaO_2 due to ventilation perfusion mismatch at the bases. Later, hypoventilation results in hypercapnoea. Finally, cor pulmonale develops in response to pulmonary hypertension. Investigation includes plain X-rays to demonstrate the angle of the scoliosis (correlates well with severity of reduction in lung volumes) and lung function testing to assess the restrictive defect. Overnight O_2 saturation monitoring assesses the degree of hypoxia.

Treatment involves monitoring for complications and treating as appropriate with the eventual need for corrective orthopaedic surgery in a number.

Prognosis depends on the cause. Idiopathic scoliosis usually has a good outcome; outcome of scoliosis due to other causes depends on the prognosis of the underlying condition.

STRIDOR

It is just possible that you might see a child with stridor. Stridor is a 'crowing' inspiratory noise due to upper airway obstruction.

INSTRUCTION

Look at this child's chest and tell me what you see and hear, what is the most likely reason for this?
What investigations are appropriate?

Case – 2-month-old infant

John is a well looking infant who looks well grown for his age although I would like to plot him on a growth chart. There is audible stridor with slight sternal recession. There is no tachypnoea. There are no scars. Chest expansion looks normal and there is no abnormality on auscultation. (Ask mother about feeding.) He is currently feeding without any problems. The most likely diagnosis is laryngomalacia, but I would also consider the following in my differential diagnosis...

NOTES ON STRIDOR

The commonest cause of stridor is laryngomalacia or 'floppy larynx', usually a benign condition that presents soon after birth. It is characteristically better when the child is laid prone. It normally has a benign course and resolves by 18 months.

Other causes to exclude

- In a sick pyrexial child – acute epiglottitis, bacterial tracheitis, severe croup
- Inhaled foreign body

- Prolonged neonatal intubation
- Vascular ring (double aortic arch, pulmonary sling or aberrant subclavian artery)
- Pierre-Robin sequence
- Tracheo/bronchomalacia
- Intraluminal web or haemangioma
- Lymphoma
- Branchial/thyroglossal cyst
- Cystic hygroma

Investigations

In children with laryngomalacia in whom a confident diagnosis can be made and there are no complications (e.g. failure to thrive, apnoea, respiratory distress) no investigations are required. In children in whom there is doubt about the diagnosis or an underlying cause is suspected then fibreoptic laryngoscopy should be performed with a barium swallow to exclude a vascular ring.

MISCELLANEOUS NOTES

ENLARGED TONGUE

Causes

- Hypothyroidism
- Mucopolysaccharidoses/GMI gangliosidosis
- Congenital hypothyroidism
- Trisomy 21
- Pseudomacroglossia
- Beckwith-Wiedemann syndrome

PIERRE-ROBIN SEQUENCE

This sequence is caused by posterior attachment of the tongue (genioglossus) together with a small mandible. This results in glossoptosis and pseudomacroglossia. The tongue commonly falls back and obstructs the airway. There is sometimes a cleft palate in addition. The mandible usually grows sufficiently within six months, but some children with severe recurrent obstruction will need either a nasopharyngeal airway or tracheostomy whilst this occurs.

TRACHEOSTOMY

Indications

- Subglottic stenosis (high tracheostomy)
- Prolonged intubation
- Severe gastro-oesophageal reflux
- Irradiation
- Neuromuscular weakness
- Severe sleep apnoea

Complications

- Hypoxia
- Arrhythmias (during suctioning)
- Decannulation
- Ulceration
- Infection
- Bleeding
- Obstruction

YOUR NOTES

CHAPTER 3 – GASTROENTEROLOGY AND HEPATOLOGY

This chapter contains information on the examination of the gastrointestinal system. Abdominal examination includes splenomegaly. Some of the causes of splenomegaly are discussed in the haematology chapter, others in this chapter. We have tried to avoid duplication. We have included a detailed review of nutritional assessment and supplementation. This can be applied to any pathology, whether gastrointestinal or related to disease in another system.

The conditions listed in this chapter are the gastrointestinal and hepatology cases likely to be seen as short cases in the exam.

SUMMARY
- ❏ Scheme for examination of the gastrointestinal system
- ❏ Abdominal scars
- ❏ Assessment of nutritional status
- ❏ Nutritional supplementation
- ❏ Gastrostomy tube feeding
- ❏ Cystic fibrosis
- ❏ Crohn's disease
- ❏ Coeliac disease
- ❏ Constipation
- ❏ Umbilical hernia
- ❏ Hepatomegaly and splenomegaly
- ❏ Examination of the liver, spleen and kidneys
- ❏ Hepatomegaly
- ❏ Glycogen storage disease
- ❏ Splenomegaly
- ❏ Portal hypertension
- ❏ Cirrhosis and liver transplantation
- ❏ Extra-hepatic biliary atresia
- ❏ Ascites

SCHEME FOR THE EXAMINATION OF THE GASTROINTESTINAL SYSTEM

Find your own system with which you are comfortable. The following is a suggested scheme.

Position the child correctly and maintain good eye contact.

Inspection – ensure adequate exposure

- Does the child look well
- Normal or dysmorphic
- Nasogastric tube, i.v. cannula
- Well nourished (adequate exposure) – comment on nutritional status
- Mention the need to plot on a growth chart
- Xanthoma

Hands

- Clubbing (causes)
- Koilonychia
- Palmar erythema
- Pallor

Eyes

- Jaundice
- Anaemia
- Blue sclera

Mouth

- Pigmentation – Peutz-Jeghers
- Mouth ulceration
- Tongue – stomatitis
- Teeth

Chest

- Spider naevi
- Gynaecomastia

Abdomen

- Scars (laparoscope, groin, loin)
- Umbilical hernia
- Abnormal vessels – caput medusae (drain from the umbilicus)
- Distension
- Superficial palpation – all over once
- Deep palpation – all over once
- Liver
- Spleen
- Kidneys

FURTHER EXAMINATION

This should be done as appropriate and depends on the previous findings. For example it is not necessary to look for shifting dullness if the abdomen is not distended.

- Percussion
- Bowel sounds
- Abdominal distension – stand child up and look at buttocks as may also be wasted suggesting malabsorption
- Ascites – fluid thrill, shifting dullness – only if distended
- Can I see the back?
- Can I see the genitalia?
- Hernia orifices

NOTES ON EXAMINATION OF GASTROINTESTINAL SYSTEM

- Xanthoma may be present and suggest a raised cholesterol as in cholestasis. They are usually on the extensor surfaces, and occasionally around the eyes.
- Mouth – large tongue – think of Down's syndrome, Beckwith-Wiedemann syndrome
- Iron deficiency anaemia – pale, blue sclera, koilonychia
- Teeth should be looked at carefully as they are a good indicator of general nutrition. Dental caries predominant at the back occurs in gastro-oesophageal reflux and at the front with poor diet – such as prolonged bottle feeding with sugary drinks.

ABDOMINAL SCARS

Case – 6-year-old boy

INSTRUCTION

Examine this child's abdomen

> The only abnormality is a scar in the right loin, the rest of the examination is normal.

- What do you think the scar may be due to?

Possible explanation would be a nephrectomy scar, the child having undergone a nephro-uretectomy because he had a cystic dysplastic kidney and there was reflux up to it. The indications for the nephrectomy would be firstly the risk of infection as a consequence of the reflux and secondly the risk of hypertension in adult life.

NOTES ON ABDOMINAL SCARS

An abdominal scar would not be an uncommon way to begin a short case. The more common childhood surgical conditions and the position of the scars associated with the surgery are listed. It is important during your revision to look at scars, to understand the possible procedures which may have resulted in that scar and to be able to talk about them.

Laparotomy scar

The finding of a laparotomy scar could incorporate a whole host of intra-abdominal pathology, but look for surrounding clues that might lead you to the diagnosis.

- Down's syndrome baby with a laparotomy incision, look for the site of a colostomy on the abdomen, and think of Hirschsprung's disease, alternatively if there is a laparotomy scar and no colostomy scar there may have been an atresia.
- Are there any signs of cystic fibrosis, and could this be a meconium ileus repair?
- Could this be an ex-premature infant who had necrotising enterocolitis during the neonatal period?

- Is there an associated thoracolumbar incision suggesting a renal transplant (feel for mass in right iliac fossa as this is the site of implantation of the donor kidney)?
- Other possibilities are Kasai procedure for biliary atresia, malrotation, intussusception, tumours, amongst others.

Kocher's incision below the right subcostal margin allows access to the liver and the biliary tree. This should alert you to the possibility of a cholecystectomy and hence look for signs of a haematological disorder such as sickle cell disease, leading to the formation of gallstones or hereditary spherocytosis.

Transverse upper abdominal incision is the site of repair of a congenital diaphragmatic hernia more common on the left than the right.

Upper abdominal midline incision think Nissen's fundoplication – is this child handicapped, is there an associated gastrostomy scar?

Small right upper transverse rectus cutting incision is the site of Ramstedt's pyloromyotomy, more common in boys.

Right iliac fossa scar could be the site of an appendectomy.

Lateral thoracolumbar incision – nephrectomy – this is commonly performed in children with cystic dysplastic kidneys to prevent infection in a redundant kidney and the development of hypertension in adult life.

Sub-umbilical/umbilical scar – suggests gastroschisis or exomphalos, again think of associated conditions. Alternatively could be an umbilical hernia repair.

Groin scars suggest inguinal hernia repair, more common in ex-premature infants.

Laparoscopy scars are frequently seen. Laparoscopic surgery is becoming more common. Scar sites are usually small and multiple.

ASSESSMENT OF NUTRITIONAL STATUS

The assessment of nutritional status is very important and can be applied to the short case examination of many systems or as a question in its own right. The information in this section is to help with that. Firstly the general case and appropriate comments are considered then specific scenarios with notes on how to deal with them.

General case

- Look at this 10-year-old boy and comment on his nutritional status

John is comfortable at rest. He looks thin. I would like to plot him on a growth chart. His muscle bulk is poor with a reduced midarm circumference and his subcutaneous fat mass is poor with a reduced skin fold thickness. I note he has a gastrostomy tube in situ. I would like to proceed with a full examination. He looks pale...

Specific scenarios arise within the different systems and need to be considered

- This 6-month-old infant has congenital heart disease – comment on his nutritional status. What nutritional supplementation would you recommend?
- This 6-month-old infant has bronchopulmonary dysplasia and severe failure to thrive. Comment on possible causes.
- This 13-year-old boy has cerebral palsy. Comment on his nutritional status. What strategies could be used to improve his nutritional status? Why do you think his nutritional status is so poor?
- This boy has cystic fibrosis and is malnourished. Comment on the cause of it. What can be done to help?

These scenarios are considered in detail later.

NOTES ON NUTRITIONAL ASSESSMENT

This is an essential part of the general examination of a patient and applicable to children with pathology from the gastrointestinal or other systems. Commenting on nutritional status is all part of making a general comment about a patient. If the nutrition looks poor then the following scheme may be helpful.

Scheme

- Obvious pathology e.g. cystic fibrosis
- Carefully plotted height, weight and head circumference
- Triceps and sub-scapular skinfold thickness
- Midarm circumference
- Presence of nasogastric tube, gastrostomy
- Nails (koilonychia)
- Pallor – hands, mucous membranes, skin
- Hair – thinning
- Pubertal status, if older

Notes

If in any doubt about nutritional status it is sensible to suggest to the examiner that you would plot the child onto a height and weight chart. The midarm circumference gives an impression about muscle bulk. The skin fold thickness gives an impression of the subcutaneous fat mass.

It is important to consider the nutritional status of patients seen. It is useful to give some thought to potential mechanisms as poor nutrition is frequently multifactorial. Cystic fibrosis provides the best example and is the most commonly seen in the exam. Others include congenital heart disease, bronchopulmonary dysplasia, severe neurological handicap and chronic inflammatory bowel disease.

Pathogenesis of malnutrition

It is essential to think about the pathogenesis of malnutrition when assessing nutrition and looking at nutritional supplementation. We can look at cystic fibrosis as an example.

The aetiology of malnutrition is often complex and various factors play a role:

1. Malabsorption causing increased losses

2. Increased energy needs

Chronic cough
Dyspnoea   } causing increased needs
Recurrent infection
Inflammation

3. Reduced intake

Anorexia
Vomiting   } resulting in reduced intake
Psychological problems

All these together result in an energy deficit. All factors need to be taken into account when nutritional supplementation is considered.

NUTRITIONAL SUPPLEMENTATION

Nutritional supplementation should be done with the help of a dietician.

Using the scenarios listed previously.

The help of a paediatric trained dietician is essential

Case 1

This 6-month-old infant has congenital heart disease – comment on his nutritional status. What nutritional supplementation would you recommend?

In this infant the poor nutritional state will be as a consequence of increased metabolic demands and poor intake secondary to breathlessness. Supplementation would be by increasing the calorie density of feeds and consideration of other methods of administration such as a nasogastric tube.

Case 2

This 6-month-old infant has bronchopulmonary dysplasia and severe failure to thrive. Comment on possible causes.

In this infant the above applies. In addition other factors may be relevant such as gastro-oesophageal reflux. Supplementation would be by increasing calorie density and considering using a nasogastric tube. In addition investigation for problems like gastro-oesophageal reflux may be considered.

Case 3

This 13-year-old boy has cerebral palsy. Comment on his nutritional status. What strategies could be used to improve it and why do you think it is so poor?

This child's principal problem will be with intake, either because of reflux or secondary to the bulbar problems or both. In addition to nutritional supplements this child may benefit from help with feeding practices including the involvement of a communication therapist and occupational therapist. Other medical problems may be relevant. Consideration needs to be given to nasogastric tube or gastrostomy tube feeding if appropriate. In some instances a fundoplication will also be required.

Case 4

This boy has cystic fibrosis and is malnourished. Comment on the cause. What can be done to help?

The additional factor in this child is malabsorption for which pancreatic supplementation is required. Children with cystic fibrosis often dislike food and need either a nasogastric tube or gastrostomy to help with administration. The energy requirements are high and calorie supplementation with energy dense supplements is required

NOTES ON NUTRITIONAL SUPPLEMENTATION
Basic information

- Normal birth weight for term infants in the UK is 3.3–3.5 kg for both sexes
- Loss of weight in first 5–7 days, then regain birth weight within the next 14 days
- Thereafter average weight gain is
  - 200 g/week for first 3 months
  - 150 g/week for second 3 months
  - 100 g/week for third 3 months
  - 50–75 g/week for fourth 3 months

Supplementation

- Nutritional supplements are generally required for those infants who are failing to thrive on normal feeds or who are fluid restricted
- Care needs to be taken not to present too high an osmotic load as osmotic diarrhoea may result

Carbohydrate supplements

- Glucose polymers are used, examples include Caloreen, Maxijul, Polycal (all hydrated cornstarch)

Fat supplements

- Usually long chain fat emulsions, examples include Calogen, Liquigen
  - Calogen   arachis oil
  - Liquigen   MCT oil

Combined carbohydrate and fat supplements
- Duocal which includes cornstarch, maize oil and coconut oil

Protein supplements
- Whole protein, peptides or amino acids
- Rarely required without an accompanying increase in other energy sources
- Examples include Maxipro HBV which is whey protein

Concentrating infant feeds
- Provide feeds more dense in energy and protein, and have the advantage of providing this without the need to add a series of supplements
- Most normal baby milks are made up to 13%, providing 65 kcal per 100 ml and protein content 1.5 g/100 ml. Making a feed up to 15% provides 75 kcal/100 ml and 1.7 g/100 ml of protein
- Carbohydrate and fat can still be added if required

GASTROSTOMY TUBE FEEDING

It is essential to have seen and to recognise a gastrostomy tube. They are generally inserted endoscopically (percutaneous endoscopic gastrostomy) and the complications are few.

Indications
- In chronic disease with nutritional impairment e.g. cystic fibrosis, bronchopulmonary dysplasia
- For nutritional therapy e.g. Crohn's disease
- Because of difficulties with feeding e.g. cerebral palsy, particularly with an associated bulbar palsy
- In severe gastro-oesophageal reflux with a fundoplication
- Children dependent upon nasogastric feeding for any other reason

**Gastrostomy tube plus transverse abdominal incision
= gastrostomy plus Nissen's fundoplication**

CYSTIC FIBROSIS

Case – 12-year-old-boy

Peter is a thin looking boy and I would like to plot him on a growth chart. He has reduced subcutaneous fat and muscle bulk. There is a gastrostomy tube in situ. He is clubbed, tachypnoeic and there is a Harrison's sulcus. Examination of his abdomen reveals hepatomegaly which is firm in consistency. There is splenomegaly and caput medusae...

I suspect he has cystic fibrosis complicated by liver disease – presumably cirrhosis associated with portal hypertension...

Case – 10-year-old girl

Sarah is a well looking caucasian girl. I would like to plot her growth parameters. She is clubbed. She has a hyperexpanded chest. On examination of the abdomen there is a transverse incision. She also has a palpable mass in the right iliac fossa.

I wonder if she has cystic fibrosis and distal intestinal obstruction syndrome...

GASTROINTESTINAL MANIFESTATIONS OF CYSTIC FIBROSIS
Pancreatic
- Insufficiency occurs in up to 90%
- Pancreatitis
- Abnormal glucose tolerance in up to 10% by the second decade
- Diabetes mellitus

Intestinal
- Meconium ileus
- Atresias
- Rectal prolapse
- Distal intestinal obstruction syndrome
- Strictures secondary to high dose pancreatic supplementation

Hepatobiliary

- Cholestasis in infancy
- Fatty liver
- Focal biliary fibrosis
- Multilobular cirrhosis
- Abnormalities of the gall bladder
- Cholelithiasis
- Obstruction of the common bile duct

CROHN'S DISEASE

This may be seen as a long or a short case or a viva topic and therefore a good knowledge base of the various aspects is required. The clinical signs are not particularly specific but an illustrative case is included.

Case – 14-year-old boy

This 14-year-old boy looks pale and thin. I suspect he is short and would like to plot him on a growth chart. His muscle bulk and subcutaneous fat mass are poor. I would like to look in his mouth for gum hyperplasia and aphthous ulceration. There is mild right iliac fossa tenderness but no other abnormalities on abdominal examination.

- I would like to check his pubertal status
- I would like to examine his peri-anal region for skin tags, fissures and fistula

There may also be

- Nasogastric tube or gastrostomy
- Signs of steroid toxicity
- Scars from previous surgery

NOTES ON CROHN'S DISEASE

Crohn's disease is a chronic inflammatory disorder of bowel involving any region from mouth to anus. The inflammation is transmural with skip lesions. There has been an increase in incidence over the past 10 years. The commonest presenting symptoms are abdominal pain, diarrhoea and weight loss although other symptoms and extra-intestinal manifestations do occur. Growth failure with delayed bone maturation and delayed sexual development is common. The aetiology of this is complex and includes poor nutritional state, disease activity, endocrine disturbance and the side-effect of corticosteroids when used. The diagnosis is made on the basis of clinical symptoms, raised inflammatory indices and diagnostic test including barium radiology and colonoscopy with biopsy. Treatment is difficult as the disease often runs a chronic relapsing course. The aim of treatment is to induce a disease remission and facilitate normal growth and development.

The most widely used treatment in children is enteral nutrition used as an exclusion diet for up to eight weeks followed by a period of controlled food reintroduction. This induces remission in up to 90% of patients. Maintenance is with 5 ASA derivatives. Unfortunately, disease relapse is common and either repeated courses of enteral nutrition or corticosteroids are required. Corticosteroid dependence or resistance can occur and additional immunosuppression or surgery may be necessary.

COELIAC DISEASE

This may be seen as a long or a short case or a viva topic and therefore a good knowledge base of the various aspects is required.

INSTRUCTION

Examine this child. Suggest a diagnosis.

Clinical features

- Often short
- Pale
- Thin with reduced subcutaneous fat, poor muscle bulk and buttock wasting
- Abdominal distension

Case

I saw a 2-year-old girl. She looks pale and is thin. I would like to plot her on a growth chart. Her muscle bulk and subcutaneous fat mass are reduced. Abdominal examination is unremarkable apart from marked distension. On standing, her distension increases and I can see buttock wasting. I suspect she has a malabsorption syndrome. Coeliac disease would be the most likely...

Supplementary questions

- What are the investigations?
- What is the management?
- What are the indications for a gluten challenge?

NOTES ON COELIAC DISEASE

Prevalence is 1 in 2000. Associations are with HLA B8, DR7, DR3 and DQw2. There is an increased incidence in first degree relatives. The intolerance is to gluten which is present in wheat, rye, barley and oats. Coeliac disease usually presents after 6 months of age (i.e. after gluten has been introduced into the diet) with chronic diarrhoea and poor weight gain. Other features include anorexia, lethargy, generalised irritability, abdominal distension and pallor. Older children may present with non-specific gastrointestinal symptoms, iron deficiency or short stature. Diagnosis is by small bowel biopsy (endoscopic duodenal or jejunal). The characteristic features on biopsy are of sub-total villous atrophy, crypt hypertrophy, intra-epithelial lymphocytes and a lamina propria plasma cell infiltrate. It is of crucial importance that the child's gluten intake is adequate at the time of the biopsy. Treatment is with a gluten free diet for life. There is a long term risk of small bowel lymphoma if the diet is not adhered to. The gluten free diet itself has no long term complications.

The standards for the diagnosis of coeliac disease are set out by the European Society of Paediatric Gastroenterology. Diagnosis is confirmed by characteristic histology and a clinical remission on a gluten free diet. There are indications for a subsequent gluten challenge and these include initial diagnostic uncertainty and when the diagnosis is made under the age of two years. The latter is because at that age there are other causes of a flat jejunal biopsy such as cows' milk protein sensitive enteropathy.

A gluten challenge involves an initial control biopsy on a gluten free diet followed by a period on gluten with a repeat biopsy after 3–6 months and then again after 2 years, sooner if symptoms develop. There are reports of late relapse following gluten challenge. Antibody testing in the screening of children with failure to thrive and in the ongoing management of children with coeliac disease is helpful. The most widely used antibody test is the IgA anti-endomysial. False negatives are seen in children who are IgA deficient.

The associations of coeliac disease are increased incidence of small bowel malignancy, especially lymphoma, increased incidence of IgA deficiency, increased incidence of autoimmune thyroid disease, pernicious anaemia and diabetes mellitus (HLA B8 associations) and dermatitis herpetiformis.

The differential diagnosis of coeliac disease is important.

Differential diagnosis of the 'malabsorptive' picture (= malabsorption syndrome)

- Coeliac disease
- Cows' milk protein intolerance
- Cystic fibrosis
- Immunodeficiency
- Others = many e.g. infection, giardiasis, soya intolerance, autoimmune disease etc.

CONSTIPATION

This has been a common short case in the last few exams

Case

This 9-year-old girl looks well. I would like to plot her on a growth chart...proceed through examination...She has a full abdomen with a palpable mass arising from the pelvis. This is hard and indents. I suspect it is faeces and that she has chronic constipation with a megarectum. I would like to examine her peri-anal region as she may have overflow soiling and it is essential to exclude local pathology such as a fissure.

NOTES ON CONSTIPATION

Most children with constipation do not have an underlying cause and their constipation is functional. If associated with a megarectum then soiling is common. This should be distinguished from encopresis in which stool is passed in to the pants at inappropriate times and in inappropriate places with no underlying constipation – the latter being a primarily psychological problem.

Underlying causes which need to be considered for the purpose of the exam
- Hirschsprung's disease
- Thyroid disease
- Meconium ileus equivalent

Hirschsprung's disease is very rare in children who have at some stage of their life had a normal bowel habit and usually presents in the neonatal period.

The management of chronic functional constipation is multidisciplinary. Many factors are often involved including local pathology such as anal fissure, poor diet, poor fluid intake, previous difficult toileting experiences and psychosocial problems. Drugs used include stimulant and bulk laxatives. Enema therapy which can reinforce difficult toileting experiences should be reserved for the more difficult cases.

UMBILICAL HERNIA

QUESTION

This 18-month-old infant has a large irreducible umbilical hernia. Does it need surgery?

NOTES ON UMBILICAL HERNIA

A common condition, presents in infancy. Almost never obstructs. Usually resolves by age two. If it has not resolved by then it is unlikely to and therefore surgery should be considered, preferably before school age.

Associated conditions
- Hypothyroidism
- Storage disorders e.g. mucopolysaccharidoses
- Beckwith-Wiedemann syndrome
- Trisomy 18
- Trisomy 13

HEPATOMEGALY AND SPLENOMEGALY

Cases likely to be seen in the exam

Hepatomegaly, splenomegaly and hepatosplenomegaly are frequently encountered in short cases. It is important to have wide differential diagnosis, however, likely causes are asked for in the patients you have seen and these should be focused on.

Hepatomegaly

- Glycogen and other storage disorders
- Right-sided heart failure

Splenomegaly

- Portal hypertension
- Idiopathic thrombocytopenic purpura
- Myeloproliferative disease
- Hereditary spherocytosis
- Sickle cell disease
- Infection – glandular fever

Hepatosplenomegaly

- Congenital hepatic fibrosis
- Cystic fibrosis
- Thalassaemia
- Mucopolysaccharidoses

EXAMINATION OF THE LIVER, SPLEEN AND KIDNEYS

- Important to do correctly
- Liver/spleen – start in right iliac fossa
- If organomegaly found confirm with percussion – measure if appropriate

Liver

- Edge – regular or irregular
- Surface – smooth or nodular
- Texture – firm or hard
- Tenderness
- Is there a rub?
- Is there a bruit?

Spleen

- As above
- ? Hepatomegaly and ascites
- Associations e.g. jaundice – hereditary spherocytosis

Common exam questions

- How do you differentiate between a liver, spleen and kidney?
- Why is it a liver?
- Why is it a spleen?

These are straightforward but commonly asked questions which are often answered badly. If you find organomegaly it is important that you assess its character carefully and make it clear to the examiner using the criteria below that you are demonstrating a liver, spleen or kidney.

Liver

- Right hypochondrium
- Cannot get above it
- Moves with respiration
- Dull to percussion

Spleen

- Left hypochondrium
- Cannot get above it
- Moves with respiration
- Dull to percussion
- Has a notch

Kidney

- Can get above it
- Doesn't move with respiration
- Resonant
- Ballotable

HEPATOMEGALY

INSTRUCTION

Examine this child's gastrointestinal system. Talk me through your examination.

Case

This is a 10-year-old girl. She looks well. She appears small. I would like to plot her on a height and weight chart (proceed to examine – lift hand). There is no evidence of clubbing or palmar erythema. (Her facies are a little immature – may or may not notice.) (Assess conjunctiva.) There is no pallor or jaundice. Her mouth looks clear with no aphthous ulceration or stomatitis. There are no spider naevi on the chest. Her abdomen is full. There are no scars or abnormal vessels. (Palpate – superficial then deep palpation – should at this stage be able to feel the large liver, then assess formally.) She has a large liver palpable in the right hypochondrium. The liver is hard and measures 6 cm below the costal margin (percuss to confirm upper border). (Feel for spleen.) There is no associated splenomegaly. Kidneys are impalpable (occasionally may be). (If clear about findings can stop there.)

In summary this is a well 10-year-old girl. She has massive hepatomegaly but no other signs of liver disease. I suspect she may have glycogen storage disease type one.

NOTES ON HEPATOMEGALY

You may be asked for a full differential diagnosis of hepatomegaly in which case you will need to have one available. We have included one. Avoid mentioning rarities and give just one or two examples in each category. You don't want to be mention some rare differential you don't know much about and then be asked about it by the examiner – black hole!! The most likely scenario is that you will be asked for a diagnosis which would be appropriate in the child you have seen. This is very important. For example you would not expect to be taken to see a child who was jaundiced with a large tender liver and infective hepatitis. Equally, one would not expect to be asked to palpate the liver of a child with extensive metastases. You are more likely to see a stable and well child with a glycogen storage disease or other storage disorder, or a child with portal hypertension or a stable child post Kasai procedure for biliary atresia. This means you need to ensure you give an appropriate and relevant answer to the questions asked and remember that many causes of organomegaly in the abdomen are not likely to be used as short cases for the exam.

There may be no physical signs in a child with liver disease such as chronic hepatitis B infection.

NOTES ON GLYCOGEN STORAGE DISEASE TYPE ONE – VON GIERKE'S DISEASE

- Autosomal recessive inheritance
- Due to reduced glucose 6 phosphatase activity
- Most common glycogen storage disease seen
- Usually presents within the first 6 months with hypoglycaemia or asymptomatic hepatomegaly
- Fasting hypoglycaemia – no response to glucagon
- Doll's face facies
- Often short with reduced intellectual development
- Large liver and occasionally large kidney
- Hepatomegaly is due to the accumulation of glycogen and fat
- At risk of hypoglycaemia and lactic acidosis – need overnight glucose infusions and frequent feeds when unwell
- Older children use corn starch which is slow release carbohydrate
- Long term risk of renal calculi and hepatoma

NOTES ON OTHER STORAGE DISEASES

Glycogen storage disease type III

- Debranching enzyme deficiency (liver and muscle)
- Massive hepatomegaly
- Myopathy
- Developmental delay
- Can progress to cirrhosis

Glycogen storage disease type IV

- Rapidly progressive hepatic disease with hepatomegaly, ascites and portal hypertension leading to cirrhosis

Glycogen storage disease type V

- Muscle only
- Poor prognosis

Gaucher's disease

- Autosomal recessive
- Deficiency in glucosylceramide beta glucosidase (glucocerebrosidase) resulting in lipid accumulation in reticuloendothelial cells
- Different forms – infant, juvenile and adult
- Can progress to portal hypertension and cirrhosis

DIFFERENTIAL DIAGNOSIS OF HEPATOMEGALY

Infection

- Hepatitis A
- Hepatitis B
- EBV infection

Storage disorders

Fat

- Cystic fibrosis
- Obesity
- Malnutrition
- TPN

Lipid

- Gaucher's disease

Glycogen

- Glycogen storage disease

Infiltration

- Primary liver tumours
- Secondary tumour e.g. lymphoma, leukaemia, neuroblastoma

Obstructive

- Hepatic vein thrombosis
- Congestive cardiac failure

Miscellaneous

- Wilson's disease
- Alpha 1 antitrypsin deficiency
- Congenital hepatic fibrosis

Idiopathic

VERY LARGE LIVER

- Storage disorder
- Reticuloendothelial disease e.g. leukaemia
- Gross fatty change
- Malignancy
- Congestive cardiac failure

SPLENOMEGALY

INSTRUCTION

Examine this child. Suggest a likely diagnosis. What are the complications?

Case

Callum is a 10-year-old boy who appears well grown. He is pale. Caput medusae are visible. His abdomen is full but not distended and he has a large spleen extending to 6 cm below the costal margin. Ascites is also present. No other signs...

Likely diagnosis: portal hypertension secondary to pre hepatic portal vein obstruction

NOTES ON SPLENOMEGALY

The aetiology of splenomegaly can be split

- Hyperplasia of the reticuloendothelial system
  - excessive antigenic stimulation – infection
  - disorders of immunoregulation – auto-immune disease
  - excessive destruction of blood cells – haemolytic anaemia
- Neoplasia
- Disorders of splenic flow – portal hypertension
- Infiltration – metabolic lesions
- Extra medullary haemopoiesis

DIFFERENTIAL DIAGNOSIS OF SPLENOMEGALY

Infection

- Bacterial, viral or protozoal
- Septicaemia
- Infectious mononucleosis
- Malaria

Autoimmune disease

- Juvenile chronic arthritis
- SLE

Haemolytic disorders

- Hereditary spherocytosis
- Sickle cell anaemia (early)

Neoplastic

- Acute leukaemia
- Hodgkin's disease

Disordered splenic flow

- Portal hypertension
- Cirrhosis
- Cardiac failure

Infiltration

- Gaucher's disease

Extra medullary haemopoiesis

- Thalassaemia

Hepatospleenogely

Infection : CMV, Hepatitis, Rubella

Hematological – Thal, sphero

Metabolic –

NOTES ON PORTAL HYPERTENSION

The cardinal feature of portal hypertension is splenomegaly. Portal hypertension does not necessarily imply liver disease. If there are no clinical or biochemical features of liver disease and the liver is not enlarged, portal vein obstruction is the most likely diagnosis. If the liver is large and there are no stigmata of cirrhosis then congenital hepatic fibrosis should be considered.

Clinical features of portal hypertension

- Splenomegaly
- Cutaneous porto-systemic shunts (caput medusae – flow from the umbilicus, venous hum above the umbilicus, haemorrhoids)
- Ascites, hypoalbuminaemia, increased incidence of infections
- Liver small, normal size or enlarged
- Failure to thrive, reduced muscle bulk

As a consequence of the portosystemic shunts, gastrointestinal haemorrhage (oesophageal varices, internal haemorrhoids) and encephalopathy.

As a consequence of the large spleen (hypersplenism)
- Thrombocytopenia
- Anaemia
- Leukopenia

Commonest causes of portal hypertension

- Cirrhosis
- Portal vein obstruction
- Congenital hepatic fibrosis
- Hepatic vein outflow obstruction

You may be asked either for the likely cause of portal hypertension in the child you see (see above) or a more comprehensive list of potential causes.

Differential diagnosis of portal hypertension

Pre hepatic
    portal vein thrombosis

Intra hepatic
    pre-sinusoidal   neoplasia
                    schistosomiasis
                    hepatic cyst
    sinusoidal   cirrhosis   biliary atresia
                                             neonatal hepatitis
                                           alpha 1 antitrypsin
                                                deficiency
    post sinusoidal   veno-occlusive disease

Post hepatic
    Budd-Chiari syndrome
    right ventricular failure
    constrictive pericarditis

Portal vein obstruction

50% no obvious aetiology, probably a developmental defect. Other causes include congenital abnormalities of the portal vein and intra-abdominal sepsis. Presentation is usually either with asymptomatic splenomegaly or life-threatening bleeding. Occasionally the presentation can be with failure to thrive.

Congenital hepatic fibrosis

Autosomal recessive. Child looks well. Large hard liver with well preserved liver function. Large spleen secondary to portal hypertension. Large polycystic kidneys (75%).

In general a child with portal hypertension in whom the underlying diagnosis is unclear would be referred to a liver centre for assessment. The main priority is the treatment of the underlying cause.

CIRRHOSIS AND LIVER TRANSPLANTATION

There are numerous disorders that can lead to cirrhosis. The most likely scenario seen will be a child with biliary atresia who has had a Kasai procedure and has progressive liver disease. Other cases can be seen but rarely. The differential diagnoses should be known and will need to be presented if a child with the stigmata of chronic liver disease/cirrhosis is seen. Remember that a cirrhotic liver is usually small.

DIFFERENTIAL DIAGNOSIS OF CIRRHOSIS

Biliary tract disorders

- Biliary atresia
- Choledochal cyst
- Congenital hepatic fibrosis
- Cystic fibrosis
- Sclerosing cholangitis

Genetic and metabolic causes

- Alpha-1 antitrypsin deficiency
- Wilson's disease
- Glycogen storage disease

Infection

- Hepatitis B and C
- CMV

Autoimmune

Drugs and toxins

- Alcohol

Nutrition

- TPN

Chronic active hepatitis refers to inflammation, necrosis and fibrosis that can lead to cirrhosis. The commonest causes are hepatitis B and C and autoimmune liver disease.

Clinical features of cirrhosis

- Failure to thrive
- Clubbing
- Anaemia
- Jaundice (variable)
- Palmar erythema
- Xanthelasma
- Spider naevi
- Large hard or small impalpable liver
- Encephalopathy

Complications of cirrhosis

- Portal hypertension
- Bleeding diatheses
- Increased susceptibility to infections
- Ascites
- Bacterial peritonitis
- Pulmonary hypertension
- Hepatoma
- Malnutrition
- Gallstone formation
- Renal failure
- Hepatic encephalopathy
- Endocrine changes
- Impaired hepatic metabolism of drugs and hormones
- Impaired neurodevelopment

Management of cirrhosis

- Determine the cause if possible and treat the underlying condition
- Minimise further liver damage
- Diet containing adequate protein and essential fatty acids, trace elements and vitamins for growth and normal activities; plus adequate calorie intake
- Ascites best dealt with by restricting salt intake and/or diuretics
- Children with alimentary bleeding should be admitted, even if small, for assessment as they may have a slow initial bleed followed by a massive bleed. Should have an IV line, and cross-match.

- Bacterial peritonitis should be managed by adequate parental education leading to early detection and then treatment with appropriate antibiotics
- Hepatic encephalopathy; prevent the accumulation of ammonia, remove/correct identifiable precipitating factors, improve liver function by reducing protein intake, antibiotics – neomycin and lactulose
- Hepatorenal failure is usually a terminal event requiring liver transplant

Liver transplantation

- Indications
  1. End stage chronic disease – likelihood of death within 12 months or evidence of deterioration which will worsen the prognosis for liver transplantation
  2. Unacceptable quality of life
  3. Fulminant or subacute liver failure – age < 2 years or INR > 4
  4. Metabolic disorders e.g. Wilson's, alpha-1 antitrypsin, galactosaemia
  5. Liver tumours

- 90% 2 year survival, 64–75% 5 year survival
- Lifelong immunosuppression
- Supply of suitable donors major limiting factor
- Can split organ between recipients or use one part of liver from a related donor

EXTRA-HEPATIC BILIARY ATRESIA – POST KASAI PROCEDURE

This is a very common short case and should be known well.

INSTRUCTION

What do you think of this girl's scar?
Examine the abdomen, what do you find, can you give a sequence of events to explain this?

Clinical findings

- Characteristic scar
- Liver may be palpable
- Signs of portal hypertension may be present
- Signs of chronic liver disease may be present

NOTES ON EXTRA HEPATIC BILIARY ATRESIA

Currently biliary atresia is the commonest indication for liver transplantation in childhood. Most of this is extra-hepatic biliary atresia. The incidence is 1 in 8000–20,000 live births. The disorder is thought to be acquired. Presents as neonatal cholestasis. Investigation is complex and any infant with prolonged jaundice which is predominantly conjugated needs to be referred to a liver centre for further assessment. Treatment is with a porto-enterostomy (Kasai procedure). The outcome is much better if surgery is carried out before 3 months of age. Post op there is a high risk of cholecystitis and children need intravenous antibiotic therapy if unwell. A proportion go on to get chronic liver disease and a number require transplantation.

NOTES ON OTHER CAUSES OF CIRRHOSIS

Intra-hepatic biliary atresia

This is less common and can be either syndromic or non-syndromic. Alagille's syndrome is an example worth remembering.

Alagille's syndrome

- Paucity of intra-hepatic bile ducts
- Characteristic facies
- Vertebral arch defects/hemivertebrae
- Growth retardation
- Mental retardation
- Hypoglycaemia
- Heart disease – usually peripheral pulmonary stenosis

Alpha-1 antitrypsin deficiency

Autosomal recessive phenotype determined by Pi (protease inhibitor) typing. The condition presents with cholestasis in infancy, cirrhosis in childhood and chronic obstructive pulmonary disease in early adult life.

Wilson's disease

Incidence is 1 in 500,000. Autosomal recessive inheritance. The pathology is as a consequence of decreased biliary excretion of copper and impaired caeruloplasmin production. Caeruloplasmin is the plasma protein which transports copper. The effects include chronic active hepatitis, portal hypertension and fulminant hepatic failure with progressive lenticular degeneration due to copper deposition. The younger children tend to present with liver disease, the adults with neurological symptoms. Kayser-Fleischer rings are seen and said to be pathognomonic. Other abnormalities include sunflower cataract, renal tubular disorders and haemolysis. The hepatic presentation can be as asymptomatic hepatomegaly, acute hepatitis, chronic active hepatitis, portal hypertension (ascites, oedema, variceal haemorrhage) or fulminant hepatic failure. The lenticular degeneration usually presents with tremor.

Diagnosis is by a low plasma caeruloplasmin level and high urinary copper excretion. The latter can occur in other forms of hepatitis and a liver biopsy is often required. In equivocal cases the increased copper excretion after chelation with D-penicillamine is of diagnostic importance. Untreated the condition is fatal. Treated the prognosis is good. Treatment is with oral penicillamine as a copper binding agent in conjunction with a low copper diet. Patients on penicillamine require vitamin B6 supplements as it is an antimetabolite.

The condition does not present under the age of 5 years.

ASCITES

QUESTION

What is ascites. How do you examine for it. What are the potential causes?

NOTES ON ASCITES

- Not obvious clinically in 50%

Clinical features

- Bulging of flanks
- Protrusion of umbilicus
- Scrotal swelling
- Fluid thrill
- Shifting dullness

Differential diagnosis is wide – four main groups of pathologies

- Cirrhosis
- Congestive cardiac failure
- Nephrotic syndrome
- Protein losing enteropathy

YOUR NOTES

YOUR NOTES

CHAPTER 4 – RENAL MEDICINE

The commonest renal case seen in the exam is nephrotic syndrome. This can occur as a long or a short case. The physical signs to elicit can either be those of nephrosis or of steroid toxicity and both should be learnt. Other renal cases are unusual. You may see a child with chronic renal failure with signs of chronic disease including short stature, nutritional impairment and pallor, who may have either a peritoneal dialysis catheter or fistula for dialysis. Children are seen post renal transplant. It is important to look for the side-effects of immunosuppression and to remember that there may be nephrectomy scars if the diseased kidneys have been removed. The transplanted kidney is likely to be in the iliac fossa and is superficial and therefore palpable.

It is important to be aware that loin scars are often seen following nephrectomy for poorly functioning dysplastic or non-functioning renal tissue in childhood. The reason for the nephrectomy being the risk of sepsis if there is ongoing reflux to the poorly functioning moiety and the long term risk of hypertension.

Renal masses are occasionally seen. The key thing is to differentiate the renal mass from a mass due to other causes e.g. spleen, faeces – and this is covered in the chapter on gastrointestinal examination. Polycystic renal disease is the most likely cause although a full differential diagnosis should be known. A large bladder would be due either to bladder outlet obstruction or a neuropathic bladder. Remember a palpable megarectum may appear to be the bladder but will indent. Prune belly syndrome may be seen and is undescended testis, abdominal wall muscle defect and muscle deficiency in the urinary system with dilation.

Measurement of blood pressure is very important and is covered in the chapter on cardiology. The underlying cause in childhood is often renal.

SUMMARY
❑ Nephrotic syndrome
❑ Steroid toxicity
❑ Renal masses
❑ Adult polycystic renal disease
❑ Beckwith-Wiedemann syndrome

NEPHROTIC SYNDROME

This is a likely case. The child may have few signs and the examiner may give you a lead such as:

INSTRUCTION

Examine this 4-year-old boy with nephrotic syndrome

> **Case**
>
> *John is four years old. He looks small for his age. I would like to plot him on a growth chart. On inspection he appears oedematous with a swollen abdomen, ankles and legs. He is a little pale. I would like to measure his blood pressure and check his peripheral perfusion. Examination of the heart...There are no pleural effusions. His abdomen is distended. There are no scars or spider naevi. There is no organomegaly. There is shifting dullness. I would like to assess his genitalia.*

I would like to test his urine
I would like to assess him for signs of steroid toxicity – see later

Supplementary questions
- How would you confirm your diagnosis?
- If he presented with abdominal pain, how would you treat him?
- Would the presence of haematuria worry you?
- What are the differential diagnoses?

NOTES ON NEPHROTIC SYNDROME

A good knowledge of nephrotic syndrome is required for all parts of the exam including a clear management plan which can be asked at any stage – the long case, the short cases or the viva. The candidate is advised to read recent review articles on the subject.

Physical signs of acute nephrotic syndrome
- Oedema
- Pallor
- Tachypnoea and dyspnoea if there is pulmonary congestion
- Pleural effusions and ascites
- Peripheral, including scrotal or vulval oedema
- Hypertension

Clinical assessment of the circulating volume

- Blood pressure and pulse
- Jugular venous pressure (difficult if oedematous)
- Core-peripheral temperature difference
- Capillary return

NB Abdominal pain is a common symptom due to splanchnic vasoconstriction as a consequence of intravascular depletion. The other cause of abdominal pain in children with nephrotic syndrome is peritonitis.

Complications of nephrotic syndrome

- Hypertension
- Acute renal failure/chronic renal failure
- Infection
- Thrombosis
- Malnutrition
- Hyperlipidaemia

Management of nephrotic syndrome

- Attention to fluid balance
- Use of human albumin solution for hypovolaemia or severe symptomatic oedema or ascites
- Steroid therapy – prednisolone 60 mg/m² until remission followed by 40 mg/m² alternate days then stop
- Treat relapses with further prednisolone
- Consider cyclophosphamide or cyclosporin for steroid dependent or steroid resistant cases

Consider referral for renal biopsy if

- Steroid resistant, i.e. does not go into remission by 28 days
- Age < 12 months or >12 years
- Persistent haematuria
- Hypertension not secondary to circulatory problems
- Renal failure

Differential diagnosis of nephrotic syndrome

- Minimal change disease – most common
- Focal segmental glomerulosclerosis
- Mesangiocapillary glomerulonephritis (also known as membranoproliferative)
- Membranous nephropathy
- Multisystem disease – Henoch-Schönlein purpura
- Systemic lupus erythematosus
- Congenital nephrotic syndrome – first 6 months

STEROID TOXICITY

> **Case** – 12-year-old boy
>
> *Jason appears short and obese and I would like to plot him on a centile chart. On general examination he has a moon face and buffalo hump. There is distension of his abdomen with striae and bruising, and he has poor muscle bulk. Jason has hirsutism and hypertrichosis, there is a central line and a naso-gastric tube in situ and a scar on his abdomen in the right groin with a palpable mass underneath it.*

These findings suggest that Jason has iatrogenic Cushing's syndrome secondary to steroid induced immunosuppression for a renal transplant. Hypertrichosis suggests he is also taking cyclosporin.

In addition I would like to measure his blood pressure and dipstick his urine for glucose.

Features of steroid toxicity (Cushing's syndrome)

- Growth retardation
- Hypertension
- Acne
- Moon face
- Buffalo hump
- Abdominal striae and bruising
- Poor muscle bulk
- Proximal myopathy
- Cataracts
- Hirsutism
- Osteopenia
- Oedema
- Psychosis
- Glycosuria

Aetiology

There are various scenarios that can lead to steroid induced toxicity that you may meet in the exam. Examples include asthma, juvenile chronic arthritis, cystic fibrosis, dermatomyositis, Crohn's disease post renal/cardiac transplant (look for relevant scars), nephrotic syndrome.

Cushing's disease is extremely rare.

RENAL MASSES

Case – 14-year-old girl
With bilateral renal masses - otherwise well. Normal blood pressure.

Suggested diagnosis: autosomal dominant polycystic renal disease

Supplementary questions
- How do you know the masses are renal – can get above it, doesn't move with respiration, resonant to percussion, ballotable
- What is the differential diagnosis?

DIFFERENTIAL DIAGNOSIS OF A RENAL MASS
- Hydronephrosis
- Cyst
- Multicystic dysplastic kidney
- Polycystic renal disease
- Wilm's tumour
- Neuroblastoma
- Compensatory hypertrophy in unilateral renal agenesis
- Renal vein thrombosis
- Storage disorder
- Beckwith-Wiedemann syndrome
- Sepsis/abscess

The investigation of choice initially is an ultrasound.

NOTES ON POLYCYSTIC RENAL DISEASE

Adult polycystic renal disease

8% of adults with chronic renal failure have autosomal dominant polycystic renal disease. Commonly presents either with an asymptomatic renal mass in late childhood or early adult life or as a consequence of complications.

Complications

- Abdominal pain
- Haematuria
- Proteinuria
- Hypertension
- Chronic renal failure

Autosomal recessive polycystic renal disease

This is much less common (1 in 40,000) presenting in the neonatal period. The prognosis is poor. Hepatic cysts are common. A number survive several years but inevitably progress to dialysis and transplantation.

NOTES ON BECKWITH-WEIDEMANN SYNDROME

A foetal overgrowth syndrome, mapped to gene locus 11p15.5. Clinically, the three major features are pre- and/or post-natal overgrowth (>90th centile), macroglossia and abdominal wall defects, with minor defects of characteristic ear signs (ear lobe creases or posterior helical pits), facial naevus flammus, hypoglycaemia, organomegaly and hemihypertrophy. The diagnosis is based on either 1) three major features; or 2) two major plus three or more minor features.

Infants are more likely to be delivered prematurely, 35% before 35 weeks. Exomphalos occurs in 50% of cases and hypoglycaemia is common which is usually mild and transient. Deaths from BWS can occur in infancy and are mainly caused by problems related to prematurity or congenital cardiac defects (<10%). During childhood, the dysmorphic features become less apparent, although the macroglossia may cause feeding problems, problems with speech and occasionally with obstructive apnoea. Surgical tongue reduction may be required in severe cases. Overgrowth is most marked in the first few years and is associated with an advanced bone age. It tends to slow down in late childhood, and most adults are <97th centile. Hemihypertrophy occurs in 25% of cases. Visceromegaly is common and neoplasia occurs in 5%, most commonly with Wilms' tumour followed by adrenocortical carcinoma, hepatoblastoma and neuroblastoma, those children with hemihypertrophy being the most at risk. By adolescence, the majority lead a normal life. There is controversy about abdominal tumour screening which some centres advocate should be by regular abdominal palpation and others by regular ultrasound examination or both.

The risk factors for Wilms' tumour are important and should be known as the association may arise as a supplementary question in a short case.

Risk factors for the development of Wilms' tumour

- Beckwith-Wiedemann syndrome
- Hemihypertrophy
- Aniridia
- DRASH syndrome

NB DRASH syndrome = ambiguous genitalia, nephropathy, Wilms' tumour

YOUR NOTES

YOUR NOTES

CHAPTER 5 – HAEMATOLOGY

Many haematological conditions are encountered during the examination of other systems.

- Skin – Purpura – Henoch-Schönlein purpura
- Joints – Swollen joint – Haemophilia
- Abdomen – Splenomegaly – Hereditary spherocytosis
- General appearance – Short stature, Malar hypertrophy – Thalassaemia

Alternatively, the examiner may be much more specific and ask for an examination of the reticuloendothelial system or for the assessment of a child with purpura. Schemes for these are given in this chapter. Individual conditions with a haematological emphasis are discussed, pointing out the key clinical features to look out for.

Splenomegaly is covered in the chapter on the examination of the gastrointestinal system.

SUMMARY

❑ Scheme for examination of the reticuloendothelial system
❑ Purpura
❑ Lymphadenopathy
❑ Hereditary spherocytosis
❑ Henoch-Schönlein purpura
❑ Thalassaemia major
❑ Sickle cell disease
❑ Miscellaneous syndromes

SOME SPECIFIC TERMINOLOGY IS USEFUL

Reticuloendothelial system

The reticuloendothelial system is the mononuclear phagocyte system and consists of cells in the bone marrow, peripheral blood and tissues highly specialised for the function of endocytosis and intracellular digestion. It plays a role in inflammation but also acts as the main line of defence against bacteria in the bloodstream and controls the haematogenous dissemination of organisms.

Hypersplenism

This is a clinical syndrome in which normal splenic function becomes excessive as the spleen and its mononuclear phagocyte tissue enlarge. The most common cause is venous obstruction such as that seen in extra-hepatic venous obstruction. Pancytopenia usually occurs.

Hyposplenism

This refers to diminished splenic function associated either with absence of the spleen (congenital or following splenectomy) or functional impairment e.g. sickle cell disease. The main consequence of hyposplenism is the risk of overwhelming bacterial septicaemia. Prophylactic penicillin and appropriate immunisation is required.

SCHEME FOR EXAMINATION OF THE RETICULOENDOTHELIAL SYSTEM

General appearance

- General state, do they look well, racial origin
- Are they well grown?
- Dysmorphology

Skin

- Pallor
- Purpura
- Central line
- Injection scars

Hands

- Should be normal – there may be pallor

Face

- Anaemia
- Jaundice
- Frontal bossing, malar prominence

Lymphadenopathy

- All areas

Abdomen

- Splenomegaly
- Hepatosplenomegaly
- Palpate both inguinal regions for lymphadenopathy
- In a male ask to palpate the testicles

LYMPHADENOPATHY

It is important to have a differential diagnosis if you find lymphadenopathy. This will depend upon whether the lymphadenopathy is localised or generalised. Cervical nodes are, for example, very common in children with either current or recurrent upper respiratory tract pathology.

- Normal nodes do not exceed 2.5 cm in diameter

Simple differential diagnosis of generalised lymphadenopathy

- Infection – infectious mononucleosis, cytomegalovirus, HIV
- Autoimmune disorders
- Leukaemia/lymphoma
- Storage diseases (rare)

PURPURA

Purpura reflects a bleeding tendency and if purpura is seen in the exam it is important to remember the differential diagnosis.

- Infection – meningococcal disease
- Thrombocytopenia – neonatal thrombocytopenia, idiopathic thrombocytopenic purpura, leukaemia
- Coagulation disturbance – disseminated intravascular coagulation, haemophilia, von Willebrand's disease
- Vasculitis – Henoch-Schönlein purpura

Children with purpura are unlikely to be acutely unwell with meningococcal disease but may be shown in the recovering phase. All children with purpura need a full systemic examination with particular focus on the reticulo-endothelial system in order to elicit a cause. In addition it is sensible to mention basic investigation which includes a full blood count, blood film and clotting screen.

Haemophilia is covered in the chapter on joints.

HEREDITARY SPHEROCYTOSIS

This is a very common short case.

> *Northern European child plus pallor, jaundice and splenomegaly =*
> *Hereditary spherocytosis until proved otherwise*

INSTRUCTIONS

Examine this child's abdomen
What is the diagnosis?
Why is he jaundiced?
This boy presents with abdominal pain, pallor and a palpable spleen.
What are your thoughts? What would you do?

Clinical findings

- Northern European child
- Looks well
- Jaundice (mild)
- Pallor
- Cholecystectomy scar (occasionally)
- Splenomegaly or splenectomy scar
- Scars may be laparoscopic

Case

This is a well looking boy. I would like to examine him. His conjunctiva are pale and he is mildly jaundiced. He has a palpable spleen. There are no other abnormalities. I suspect that he has hereditary spherocytosis...

Case

This is well looking boy. There is no pallor or lymphadenopathy. He has a cholecystectomy and splenectomy scar. Is the underlying diagnosis hereditary spherocytosis...?

NOTES ON HEREDITARY SPHEROCYTOSIS

Autosomal dominant condition. Incidence is 1 in 5000 in Northern Europeans. Usually presents in childhood with the classical triad of anaemia, jaundice and splenomegaly. The jaundice is unconjugated and worsens during infections. Pigmented gallstones are present in 85% by the second decade. Aplastic crises can occur. The diagnosis is made on clinical grounds, by observing the spherocytes on a blood film and by the increased osmotic fragility of red cells when tested. Treatment is with folic acid supplements and later by splenectomy, particularly if the haemoglobin is consistently less than 10 g/dl. Cholecystectomy is occasionally required. The spleen is the site of red cell destruction. Removal of it will reduce haemolysis and reduce the incidence of gallstones. There is however an increased risk of pneumococcal and other infection. Pneumococcal, meningococcal and haemophilus influenza type B immunisation and lifelong prophylactic penicillin need to be given.

Differential diagnosis – other causes of haemolytic anaemia include

- Hereditary elliptocytosis
- Pyruvate kinase deficiency
- Autoimmune haemolytic anaemia

HENOCH-SCHÖNLEIN PURPURA
INSTRUCTION
Look at this child's legs, what do you see?

> *Purpuric rash, limited to the extensor surfaces and buttocks, does not blanch with pressure, urticarial in places, also appears to have a swollen left ankle, not hot to touch, not red, not tender, limitation of movement in all directions. The right foot does not appear abnormal and...*

What is your diagnosis?
Henoch-Schönlein purpura

What is the differential diagnosis?
- Other vasculitis e.g. systemic lupus erythematosus
- Thrombocytopenia although this wouldn't explain the swollen joint
- Sepsis but the child does not look unwell
- Could be leukaemia

This is Henoch-Schönlein purpura. What are the features of the disease?

Features of Henoch-Schönlein purpura
- Urticarial/purpuric rash, mostly on extensor surfaces and buttocks
- Arthritis in 60–80%
- Gastrointestinal involvement – including colicky abdominal pain, vomiting, GI bleeding, intussusception, pancreatitis, occurs in 50–70%
- Renal involvement in 20–90% – including microscopic haematuria, frank haematuria and proteinuria, nephrotic/nephritic picture, renal failure and hypertension
- Neurological involvement is recognised, but usually mild
- Lung involvement is rare
- Testicular involvement may manifest as uni/bilateral orchitis

NOTES ON HENOCH-SCHÖNLEIN PURPURA

Commonest vasculitis of childhood with incidence of 14–18/100,000 children per year. 50% in children under 5 years, 75% in under 10 years. Commoner in males and in winter months. Aetiology unclear, often history of preceding viral upper respiratory tract illness. There are no specific laboratory diagnostic tests. Renal involvement is usually benign but occasionally severe with a fulminant nephrotic/nephritic picture. Treatment remains controversial. Use of steroids for abdominal pain is generally well accepted although there are concerns that steroids may mask a worsening gastrointestinal picture or a lymphoproliferative disorder. Joint symptoms should be treated as required with analgesia and rest. The treatment of renal complications requires the help of a paediatric nephrologist. All patients with significant renal involvement require long term follow up. The morbidity is principally due to renal involvement, and hence the prognosis depends on the degree of renal involvement.

THALASSAEMIA MAJOR

Thalassaemia and the different variants are often seen in the exam. If you work in a hospital where such cases are rare then it is essential to read about and try to get to see some cases as you may see them in the exam.

Clinical findings
- Mediterranean/African/Indian/SE Asian child
- Multiple IV cannula sites in the hands, may be a portacath
- Jaundice (mild), pallor
- Multiple depigmented patches on abdominal wall from subcutaneous desferrioxamine administration
- Palpable spleen

Think thalassaemia major

The above refers to a well controlled thalassaemic on a regular transfusion regime. A poorly controlled thalassaemic or someone who is well controlled now but was previously poorly controlled may have signs of extra-medullary haemopoiesis.

- Frontal bossing
- Malar hyperplasia
- Hepatomegaly
- Splenomegaly
- Previous long bone fracture sites

NOTES ON THALASSAEMIA

The thalassaemias are a heterogeneous group of recessively inherited disorders characterised by deficient synthesis of either alpha or beta chains of haemoglobin. There are various different types and there are approximately 100 different mutations known to cause thalassaemia, many of which are unique to localised geographical areas. These notes are about thalassaemia major. This occurs in the populations mentioned above and produces a severe progressive haemolytic anaemia during the second six months of life. The anaemia is microcytic and hypochromic, with poikilocytes and target cells on the peripheral blood film. There are large numbers of nucleated red cells and a marked increase in HbF. In untreated or inadequately transfused patients there is proliferation of medullary and extramedullary haemopoiesis with massive expansion of the skull and face causing characteristic facies. The spleen and liver are enlarged, the bones become weak and have pathological fractures, growth is impaired and puberty delayed, diabetes mellitus occurs due to pancreatic siderosis and cardiac failure due to cardiac siderosis. With the modern technique of management many of these complications can be avoided and others ameliorated and their onset delayed.

Treatment involves a hyper transfusion regime giving blood transfusions on a regular basis to maintain haemoglobin above 10 g/dl. Haemosiderosis is however a complication of hyper transfusion and should be prevented with desferrioxamine given as a subcutaneous infusion over an 8–12 hour period 5–6 nights per week. The injection sites give rise to the depigmented patches on dark skin that are seen in most patients. Chelation therapy should commence when the ferritin has reached 800–1000 mg/l, usually around the 12–14th transfusion. Splenomegaly may eventually occur and splenectomy may be necessary. This will often reduce the transfusion requirement but there is a high risk of bacterial sepsis. Bone marrow transplantation is considered to be curative, and is being used with increasing success. However, it carries a considerable morbidity and mortality, and currently is only used if there is a non-affected histocompatible sibling donor.

SICKLE CELL DISEASE

Like thalassaemia, sickle cell disease is commonly seen in the exam. If you work in an area where sickle cell disease is rarely seen then you need to read about and be very familiar with the condition.

> *Afro-Caribbean child with pallor, jaundice and no palpable spleen = sickle cell disease until proven otherwise.*

INSTRUCTIONS

Examine this child, what do you find. Pallor, jaundice.
What is the likely diagnosis?
Feel his abdomen what do you find? Usually normal – why can you not feel his spleen?
This child presents with a pyrexia, unwell, how would you manage him?
This child presents in acute respiratory distress, what are the possibilities and how would you manage him?
This child presents with acute abdominal pain, how would you manage him?

Clinical findings

- Afro-Caribbean child, usually appears well
- Short stature
- Jaundiced (mild), pallor
- May be cholecystectomy scar
- Splenomegaly in an infant, spleen not usually palpable in an older child
- Otherwise examination unremarkable

If acutely unwell look for

- Signs of infection
- Hydration
- Chest – sequestration
- Abdominal – acute splenic enlargement
- Joints – dactylitis

NOTES ON SICKLE CELL DISEASE

Sickle cell disease is caused by a point mutation in the beta-globin gene causing deoxygenated HbS to polymerise and distort the shape of the red blood cell, decreasing red cell lifespan. It is most common in Africa, the Mediterranean, the Middle East and India. Usually asymptomatic until 5–6 months, often acute dactylitis is the first manifestation. The problems are due either to haemolysis or vaso-occlusion. Haemolysis leads to chronic anaemia, jaundice, aplastic crises, cholelithiasis, delayed growth and sexual maturation. Vaso-occlusion causes recurrent acute pain, functional asplenia, splenic sequestration, acute chest syndrome, stroke, enuresis, papillary necrosis, avascular necrosis, proliferative retinopathy and leg ulcers. The most frequent manifestation is acute painful vaso-occlusive episodes causing severe pain sometimes requiring hospitalisation and intravenous analgesia. The quoted incidence is one per year, although patients vary, some having more episodes and some never experiencing pain. The vaso-occlusive episodes affect many organs and cause gross ischaemic damage. Young children may have splenic enlargement associated with haemolysis and progress to hypersplenism. This acute splenic sequestration can cause circulatory collapse and may require lifesaving blood transfusions. However, whether they have splenic enlargement or autosplenectomy, they all have functional asplenia and are therefore at risk of overwhelming infections from encapsulated organisms. They are also at risk of *Salmonella* osteomyelitis. In common with other patients with chronic haemolysis, patients with sickle cell disease are at risk of developing aplastic crises secondary to parvovirus infection.

Diagnosis is based on haemoglobin estimation, blood film containing target cells, poikilocytes and irreversibly sickled cells and haemoglobin electrophoresis. The Hb electrophoresis result is confirmed with a further test e.g. electrophoresis at acidic pH. Treatment is aimed at preventing serious complications. They must maintain full immunisation status and be on prophylactic penicillin from at least 3 months. They need prompt help if they become febrile with parenteral antibiotics. Painful episodes may require hospital admission. Transfusions are usually limited to those patients with disabling chronic pain, severe sickling crisis, sequestration or prior to surgery (exchange transfusion).

Hb SC disease is a milder variant with moderately severe anaemia and splenomegaly. Vaso-occlusive episodes are less frequent and usually milder. Aseptic necrosis of the femoral head is common.

MISCELLANEOUS SYNDROMES

Fanconi's anaemia

This is an autosomal recessive aplastic anaemia with a pre malignant potential. There are characteristic physical findings in 50–75%. Pancytopenia develops towards the end of the first decade.

- Short stature
- Hyperpigmentation
- Microcephaly
- Microphthalmia
- Hypoplasia/aplasia of the thumb
- Renal anomalies
- Skeletal anomalies
- Mental retardation

Diamond-Blackfan syndrome

This is a pure red cell aplasia. There are no characteristic physical findings.

Wiskott-Aldrich syndrome

- X-linked
- Severe eczema
- Thrombocytopenia
- Immunodeficiency

Thrombocytopenia absent radius (TAR) syndrome

- Autosomal recessive
- Absent radii is the most common finding
- Cardiac, renal or other skeletal malformations may occur
- High mortality from bleeding in the first year of life

YOUR NOTES

YOUR NOTES

CHAPTER 6 – THYROID DISEASE

Patients with thyroid disease are commonly seen in the exam. These patients are stable and usually well. A good scheme for the examination of the neck and thyroid status is required in addition to basic knowledge about thyroid disease.

SUMMARY

❑ Scheme for examination of the thyroid gland
❑ Scheme for examination of thyroid status
❑ Symptoms and signs of thyroid disease
❑ Thyroglossal cyst
❑ Thyroid eye disease
❑ Notes on thyroid disease
❑ Examination of the anterior neck

THYROID DISEASE
INSTRUCTIONS

Examine this child's neck.
Assess this child's thyroid status.
Look at this child's neck and tell me what you see.
This child is hyperthyroid/hypothyroid. Assess her thyroid status, what medications would you expect her to be on?

> **Case** – 12-year-old girl
>
> *Sarah is a well looking girl who appears appropriately grown for her age. I would like to plot her height and weight on a centile chart. There is an obvious goitre which moves with swallowing. It is diffusely enlarged, non-tender and firm. There is no lymphadenopathy or retrosternal extension. Sarah has proptosis. I would like to examine her thyroid status and perform pubertal staging...*

SCHEME FOR EXAMINATION OF THE THYROID GLAND

Need a glass of water (may be beside the bed)

Start by making general comments – does the child look well, do they seem appropriately grown.

INSPECTION
- From the front with the neck extended for enlargement of the thyroid gland and hearing aid (Pendred's syndrome)
- Is the enlargement uniform or unilateral, are there any scars?
- If scar present check voice for hoarseness
- Ask the child to take a drink, a thyroid swelling should move upwards with swallowing
- Ask child to stick tongue out (if rises during manoeuvre = thyroglossal cyst)

PALPATION

- Palpate the gland whilst standing behind the child
- Assess size, shape, consistency and surface of the mass (single diffusely enlarged thyroid, a single enlarged cyst or a multinodular goitre?)
- Again ask to drink whilst palpating

FURTHER EXAMINATION

- Examine tongue for high thyroglossal cyst (originates at foramen caecum)
- Palpate for lymphadenopathy
- Percuss sternum for retro-sternal extension
- Auscultate mass for bruits

To say at end of examination

I would now routinely proceed to assess the thyroid status. If you do not say this you will probably be asked to do so by the examiner – save time.

SCHEME FOR EXAMINATION OF THYROID STATUS

- Look generally at the child
- Comment on growth and pubertal status and the need to plot on growth chart
- Look at the hands for clubbing (thyroid acropachy)
- Feel hands – warm and sweaty (hyperthyroid) or cold and blue (hypothyroid)
- Ask to hold arms outstretched for fine tremor (hyperthyroid)
- Count pulse
- Take blood pressure (wide pulse pressure in hyperthyroidism)
- Examine eyes for exophthalmos and lid lag and external ophthalmoplegia
- Look in mouth (delayed dentition if hypothyroid)
- Examine cardiovascular system for flow murmurs and hyperactive precordium (hyperthyroidism)
- Tendon reflexes (hypothyroidism – slow relaxation)
- Ask to examine pubertal staging

- Occasionally get a proximal myopathy in hyperthyroidism
- Think about signs of other autoimmune diseases

SYMPTOMS AND SIGNS OF THYROID DISEASE

Symptoms of hypothyroidism

- Low energy levels
- Good schoolwork (quiet attentive pupils whose work deteriorates after treatment)
- Constipation
- Delayed puberty (a small proportion have precocious puberty)
- Delayed tooth eruption
- Increased tendency to sleep
- Cold intolerance

Symptoms of hyperthyroidism

- Anxiety
- Poor sleep
- Sweating
- Heat intolerance
- Palpitations

Questions to ask to help assess thyroid status

- Energy levels
- Schoolwork (usually well behaved if hypothyroid)
- Heat tolerance/sweatiness
- Constipation/diarrhoea
- Appetite and weight loss
- Muscle weakness

Signs of hypothyroidism

- Cold hands
- Thick skin
- Bradycardia
- Slow relaxing tendon reflexes

Signs of hyperthyroidism

- Warm sweaty hands
- Fine tremor on holding arms outstretched
- Tachycardia
- Wide pulse pressure and high systolic pressure
- Hyperactive precordium
- Exophthalmos
- Lid lag
- External ophthalmoplegia

THYROID EYE DISEASE

Signs of thyroid eye disease

- Lid oedema
- Exophthalmos/proptosis
- Lid lag (eyelid lags behind eyeball on rapid down gaze)
- Conjunctival injection and oedema
- External ophthalmoplegia

NOTES ON THYROID EYE DISEASE

Thyroid eye disease is caused by antibodies against antigens shared by the thyroid and eye muscles. Retro-orbital inflammation and oedema of the extra-ocular muscles causes exophthalmos (synonymous with proptosis) and limited eye movements. The proptosis can be permanent. Eye changes are present bilaterally but asymmetrically and commonly persist when euthyroid, and can worsen if rendered hypothyroid. The most concerning complications are exposure keratopathy (secondary to reduced blinking and being unable to fully close the eye) and optic atrophy (secondary to pressure effects behind the eye). An uncommon complication in childhood is external ophthalmoplegia, this is caused by lymphocytic infiltration and glycosaminoglycan deposition in the medial and inferior rectus muscles.

NOTES ON THYROID DISEASE

Causes of goitre

- Autoimmune thyroiditis
- Graves' disease
- Colloid/simple – normal thyroid function and no antibodies
- Hyperplasia
- Diffuse nodular non-toxic
- Sub-acute thyroiditis (inflamed gland)
- Carcinoma
- Infiltration (LCH)

EUTHYROID CAUSES OF GOITRE

The commonest cause of goitre worldwide is endemic which is secondary to dietary deficiency of iodine usually seen in developing countries. This results in compensatory hypertrophy – you are very unlikely to see this in the examination. More common in the developed world is a child with autoimmune thyroiditis who is euthyroid. Thyroid antibodies are usually present.

Simple or colloid goitres present as diffusely enlarged goitres in peripubertal girls. There are no thyroid antibodies. Multinodular goitres are rare and if seen malignancy needs to be excluded.

HYPERTHYROIDISM

Usually Graves' disease, an auto-immune disease caused by production of thyroid stimulating antibodies. Peak incidence is in adolescent girls. Family history is common, and there is an association with HLA DR3/B8.

Presentation

- Often insidious
- Emotional disturbance and motor hyperactivity
- Sweatiness and increased appetite
- Weight loss/gain
- Heat intolerance
- Deterioration in school work

Investigations

- TSH low, T4 high
- Thyroid stimulating antibodies (TSH receptor stimulating antibodies) present and disappear on remission
- Bone age advanced
- Investigate first degree relatives

Treatment

Almost half of childhood cases will remit spontaneously within 2–4 years. Many will progress to become clinically hypothyroid. Medical treatment is with carbimazole and propranolol (the latter to control acute symptoms). Block replacement means that both carbimazole and thyroxine are used. Definitive treatment (favoured by many) is either by sub total thyroidectomy or the use of radioactive iodine. Severe eye disease may require treatment with prednisolone.

CONGENITAL HYPOTHYROIDISM

Incidence 1:4000, usually asymptomatic until 6–12 weeks of age due to transplacental passage of maternal thyroid hormone.

Presentation

- Raised TSH on the Guthrie card
- Poor feeding
- Hoarse cry
- Constipation
- Lethargy
- Jaundice
- Wide fontanelles
- Macroglossia
- Umbilical hernia
- Developmental delay
- Later...typical facies

Aetiology

- Thyroid dysgenesis (90%) (1/3 aplasia, 2/3 ectopic)
- Dyshormonogenesis
- TSH/TRH deficiency – look for associated midline defects
- Transplacental anti-thyroid drugs

Treatment

This is with lifelong thyroid hormone replacement with thyroxine monitored with regular thyroid function tests. There is the occasional case of transient hypothyroidism and so usually a trial off therapy is carried out in older children.

Outcome

Early treatment results in improved intelligence. Factors of relevance are compliance and the severity of thyroid dysfunction at diagnosis (particularly the TSH).

JUVENILE (ACQUIRED) HYPOTHYROIDISM

Aetiology – depends on whether goitre present

Goitre present	No Goitre
• Auto-immune thyroiditis (commonest)	• Hypoplastic or ectopic thyroid
• Dyshormonogenesis	• Hypothalamo/hypopituitary hypothyroidism – post irradiation
• Endemic iodine deficiency	
• Goitrogen exposure	
• Infiltration	• Thyroidectomy

AUTOIMMUNE THYROIDITIS

More common in girls (5:1), onset is after 6 years, peaking in adolescence. A family history is common.

Presentation

- Goitre and growth delay commonest
- Thyroid diffusely enlarged in 2/3
- Most clinically euthyroid
- Can be hypothyroid or even hyperthyroid

Associations

- Trisomy 21, 45XO, Noonan's syndrome
- Polyglandular autoimmune disease type I
      Autoimmune thyroiditis
      Addison's disease
      Mucocutaneous candidiasis
      Hypoparathyroidism
- Polyglandular autoimmune disease type II
      Addison's disease
      IDDM
      Thyroiditis
- Pernicious anaemia, vitiligo, alopecia

Diagnosis

T4 low and TSH high but may be euthyroid at diagnosis.
Microsomal and thyroglobulin antibodies usually positive.

Treatment

T4 replacement if hypothyroid.

- Warn parents that school performance and behaviour deteriorate after starting treatment but will gradually settle down.
- Monitor T4 and TSH, modest elevations of TSH are common in the treated group and this is related to under treatment. A low TSH and normal T4 may indicate erratic medication and improved compliance just before the clinic appointment.
- Arrange a trial without treatment at some stage (usually when growth is complete) to rule out transient hypothyroidism.

THYROID CANCER

This is rare in childhood and you are unlikely to see a case but may be asked to say something about it. Thyroid cancer is strongly suggested by a solitary nodule with local lymphadenopathy which shows as a cold nodule on isotope scanning.

Types
- Benign adenomata (the most common)
- Papillary
- Follicular
- Medullary
- Undifferentiated

Diagnosis is by biopsy.

Treatment is surgical removal.

EXAMINATION OF THE ANTERIOR NECK

Remember other things can be seen on examination of the anterior neck

It is important to have a list of causes to hand as this is a very common exam scenario.

- Thyroglossal cyst
- Cystic hygroma
- Haemangioma
- Sternomastoid tumour
- Lymphadenopathy
- Branchial cyst

Case –10-year-old boy

Samuel is a well looking boy who appears appropriately grown. He has an obvious midline swelling of his neck. This is seen to rise on sticking out his tongue but not on swallowing. The mass is smooth and firm. There is no local lymphadenopathy. The most likely diagnosis is a thyroglossal cyst.

Thyroglossal cyst

This is a cyst located in the midline of the neck in the route of descent of the thyroid gland from the foramen cecum. They typically rise when the tongue is protruded. They must be differentiated from an undescended lingual thyroid by radionuclide scanning as removal of ectopic thyroid tissue may render an individual hypothyroid.

YOUR NOTES

YOUR NOTES

CHAPTER 7 – GROWTH AND PUBERTY

Assessment of growth is crucial in the exam in both the long and short cases. Remember in the long case to plot the child on the growth chart. Children with both tall and short stature are frequently seen in the exam and approach to the assessment and knowledge of the common conditions seen is required. During the short cases if you think a child is tall or short you should say so and say that you would plot them on a growth chart.

Conditions which are common in the examination

Familial short stature
Familial tall stature
Turner's/Noonan's syndrome
Achondroplasia
Systemic disease
  (e.g. cystic fibrosis)

Storage disorders (e.g. Hurler's syndrome)
Marfan's syndrome
Klinefelter's syndrome
Homocystinuria

SUMMARY

❑ Growth and puberty
❑ The short child
❑ Scheme for the examination of a short child
❑ Notes on specific conditions
❑ Tall stature
❑ Scheme for examination of a tall child
❑ Notes on specific conditions

BACKGROUND INFORMATION ON GROWTH AND PUBERTY

Phases of growth

It is important to remember the phases of growth.

- 0–1 year dependent on nutrition
- 1–6 years related to growth hormone secretion
- 6–8 years mid-childhood growth spurt, coinciding with secretion of adrenal androgens
- Puberty, gonadotrophins cause sex steroid release, this in turn causes the pulsatile release of growth hormone (GH) and the consequent growth spurt

Growth stops when the epiphyses fuse.

Puberty

In boys the first sign of puberty is growth of the testicles to 4 ml and beyond (estimated with an orchidometer). This is followed two years later by the rapid growth phase and breaking of the voice, by this time testicular enlargement and genital development are usually well advanced.

In girls the changes of puberty are approximately two years earlier, the first feature is usually breast enlargement. This is followed by pubic hair development and menstruation is relatively late, occurring after the growth spurt.

In both sexes the pubic hair is mostly caused by androgen secretion from the adrenal glands, so-called adrenarche. The sex steroids control the other sexual characteristics and are responsible for eventual fusion of the epiphyses and cessation of growth.

It is unlikely that you will be asked to stage puberty in the examination, but you will need to be familiar with the various stages and be able to describe them.

Boys

- Stage 1: Pre-adolescent childhood proportions of testes and genitals
- Stage 2:   enlargement of testes and scrotum
- Stage 3:   lengthening of penis
- Stage 4:   increased breadth of penis, development of glans penis
- Stage 5: Adult

Girls

- Stage 1: Pre-adolescent
- Stage 2:   breast bud, elevation of breast and papilla as mound
- Stage 3:   further enlargement of breast and areola, no separation
- Stage 4:   projection of areola and papilla
- Stage 5: Adult

Precocious sexual development

Remember that changes in growth are closely linked to abnormalities in the pubertal process. True precocious puberty has features of normal puberty, but occurs early. The age of 8 in girls and 9 in boys is regarded as abnormally early.

True precocious puberty is commoner in girls than in boys and is idiopathic in the majority of cases. True precocious puberty in boys is uncommon and usually pathological, over half will have some form of intra-cranial pathology. The psychological problems are significant. Most will initially be tall but will end up with a reduced final height due to premature fusion of the epiphyses.

If the full picture of puberty does not develop it is not likely to be true precocious puberty. Girls may get breast enlargement (premature thelarche) or isolated pubic hair development (adrenarche) due to increased adrenal androgens.

In boys, if the testes are enlarged then it is likely to be true precocious puberty, if there is isolated pubic hair/penile development then the source of androgen is not testicular and is most likely adrenal.

Delayed puberty

This is present if there are no signs of puberty at age 13 years in girls and 14 years in boys. In the great majority it is physiological and when the testes enlarge or the breasts develop, all can be reassured. In girls in whom there is no breast development, Turner's syndrome needs to be excluded.

THE SHORT CHILD

QUESTION

What do you think is the cause of this child's short stature?

> **Case** – 15-year-old-girl
>
> *Sarah is a well looking girl who appears short for her age and I would like to plot her height and weight on a centile chart. Examination reveals webbing of her neck and cubitus valgus. She has a short 5th metacarpal and dysplastic nails. The most likely diagnosis is Turner's syndrome. I would like to examine her cardiovascular system and stage pubertal development.*

Turner's syndrome is a straightforward case and one commonly seen. Often things are not so straightforward and if so it is often difficult to know where to begin. Try to be prepared for such a case with a structured approach.

SCHEME FOR THE EXAMINATION OF A SHORT CHILD

This is quite difficult. Below is a guide to aid your consideration of the child; it should not be interpreted too literally but adapted to the child you see.

AUXOLOGY

Offer to measure height (including sitting height if you suspect a skeletal dysplasia), weight, head circumference and if appropriate sub-scapular/triceps skinfold thickness and pubertal stage and plot on appropriate centile charts. Clearly if a short child is obviously post pubertal it is relevant and should be stated. Offer to measure parents' height.

1. Is the child obviously dysmorphic?

For example Turner's syndrome, Noonan's syndrome, Russell-Silver dwarfism, Prader-Willi syndrome, Cornelia de Lange syndrome, Rubenstein Taybi, Aarskog's, mucopolysaccharidoses. If so then direct the examination towards that problem.

2. Limb/spine proportions

Examine arms for rhizomelic (proximal), mesomelic (distal) or symmetrical shortening, a useful way to do this is to fully flex the arm at the elbow and compare upper arm with lower.

Rhizomelic shortening: Achondroplasia (frontal bossing, lordosis, etc), Rhizomelic chondrodysplasia punctata (like achondroplasia with less severe cranio-facial features)

Mesomelic shortening: mesomelic dysplasia, Ellis-van Creveld (natal teeth, hypoplastic nails, polydactyly, cardiac anomalies)

Non-rhizo/mesomelic short arms and trunk

Spondyloepiphyseal dysplasia
Hypochondroplasia (milder cranial features of achondroplasia)
Mucopolysaccharidoses (coarse facies and hepatosplenomegaly),
GM-1 (cherry red spot)

Asymmetrical limbs

Chondrodysplasia punctata
Hemi-hypertrophy, for example in Russell-Silver

Short spine only

Spinal irradiation

3. Extend arm and examine carrying angle (cubitus valgus in Turner's syndrome)

4. Examine hands for hypoplastic, hyperconvex nails (Turner's syndrome), short 5th metacarpal (Turner's syndrome and pseudohypoparathyroidism)

5. Is there an obvious systemic disease?

Thin child
- Cystic fibrosis/bronchiectasis
- Coeliac disease (wasted buttocks)
- Inflammatory bowel disease (mouth ulcers, NG tube)
- IDDM (look for lipoatrophy, lipohypertrophy)

Fat child
- Cushingoid
- Hypothyroidism (examine for goitre)
- Hypopituitarism/growth hormone deficiency

Other possibilities
- Constitutional delay
- Familial short stature
- Emotional/food deprivation

7. Ask to perform a full systemic examination

8. Discuss investigations as appropriate based on the clinical findings

Bone age

A bone age is useful. It will be delayed in constitutional delay and hormonal causes, but normal in familial short stature.

INTERPRETATION OF PARENTAL HEIGHTS AND CALCULATION OF THE EXPECTED HEIGHT

Interpreting parental height

Expected centile = (mother's height centile + father's height centile)/2

Expected final adult height

Boy (father's height + (mother's height +12.5 cm))/2

Girl ((father's height-12.5 cm) + mother's height)/2

GROWTH HORMONE

QUESTION

Which conditions are you aware of that may be treated with growth hormone?

NOTES ON GROWTH HORMONE

Biosynthetic growth hormone has been used since 1985. It acts to promote skeletal growth, lipolysis and anabolism. Side-effects of therapy include unmasking hypothyroidism, insulin resistance, slipped femoral epiphysis, GH antibodies and salt and water retention. There is no evidence of a predisposition to malignancy. Current indications for GH therapy include GH deficiency, Turner's syndrome and renal failure.

1. GH deficiency

Growth hormone is given in daily injections. There is evidence of attenuation of growth response after the first year of treatment and alteration of dose makes little difference to this. Treated children can expect to approach their target heights. Failure of treatment is usually due to poor compliance, other possibilities to consider are hypothyroidism, occult skeletal dysplasia or emotional deprivation.

2. Turner's syndrome

Most girls with this condition are short (15–20 cm below target height even with oestrogen treatment). There is an associated bone dysplasia and growth hormone resistance as well as failure of the pubertal growth spurt. Initial studies suggested an increased growth velocity in the first year of 2 cm/year more than pre-treatment velocity. Results of long term follow up are mixed.

3. Renal failure

High doses of the growth hormone result in an increase in height over two years. Long term results are awaited.

4. Other conditions

Children who are short and have no biochemical evidence of growth hormone deficiency will gain 2–3 cm in final height if treated. This does not justify its widespread use. There is no effect on constitutionally delayed puberty, nor on children with in-uterine growth retardation. There is no long term data on children with Down's syndrome, skeletal dysplasias, Prader-Willi or Noonan's syndrome. Some children with Russell-Silver dwarfism have a true GH deficiency and these will respond to replacement therapy.

TURNER'S SYNDROME

Occurs in 1:2000 female births. 50% are due to 45X0, 15% due to mosaic 45X0/46XX. Risk does not increase with maternal age.

PRESENTATION

At birth

- Lymphoedema of hands and feet
- Low posterior hairline
- Webbed neck
- Cardiac lesion (coarctation/bicuspid aortic valve)

Older child

- Delayed puberty
- Short stature
- Low hairline
- Webbed neck
- Cubitus valgus (widened carrying angle)
- Shield chest and wide spaced nipples
- Coarctation of the aorta/bicuspid aortic valve
- Horseshoe kidney
- Hyperconvex fingernails and short 4th/5th metacarpals

Cardiac lesions most commonly consist of a coarctation with a non-obstructive bicuspid aortic valve. Other possibilities include aortic stenosis and total anomalous pulmonary venous drainage. The ovaries degenerate into streaks in 90% by 10 years of age. Puberty rarely occurs though 10% may have breast enlargement. Levels of plasma gonadotrophins are markedly elevated.

30% of patients have renal anomalies, also including pelvic kidney and PUJ obstruction. Glue ear is common as is sensori-neural hearing deficit. Learning difficulties are usually mild.

Remember the associations with autoimmune disease such as autoimmune thyroiditis and inflammatory bowel disease.

NOONAN'S SYNDROME

> **Case** – 12-year-old boy
>
> *Jason is a short boy (I would like to plot his height and weight on the appropriate charts). He has hypertelorism, ptosis, micrognathia, epicanthic folds and low set ears. Examination of his chest reveals widely spaced nipples and an ejection systolic murmur grade 3/6 loudest in the pulmonary area. It does not radiate to his carotid arteries. The most likely diagnosis is Noonan's syndrome. His murmur is likely to be due to pulmonary stenosis. I would also like to examine his genitals for cryptorchidism and stage his puberty.*

NOTES ON NOONAN'S SYNDROME

A sporadic condition mapped to chromosome 12.

Presentation

- Typical facies – hypertelorism, anti-mongoloid slant, epicanthic folds, ptosis, micrognathia, low set ears
- Wide spaced nipples, cubitus valgus, short stature and pubertal delay
- Pulmonary valve stenosis, atrio-septal defect, cardiomyopathy
- Cryptorchidism, hernias

RUSSELL-SILVER DWARFISM

This is a difficult clinical diagnosis but a diagnosis that should be considered in an appropriate child.

Features

- Growth failure
- Triangular facies and frontal bossing
- Micrognathia
- Clinodactyly
- Café-au-lait spots
- Hemi-hypertrophy
- Hypopituitarism

ACHONDROPLASIA

Incidence 1:20,000, autosomal dominant 4p. Patients can expect to have a normal life span, but sudden death can occur due to cervical cord compression because of a small foramen magnum. Special height, weight, head circumference and development charts exist for the condition. Spirometry should be performed as all patients have reduced lung capacity.

If you are faced with a short child who obviously has achondroplasia, this is an approach to your examination:

- Describe the facial features to the examiner – frontal bossing, flat nasal bridge, large head circumference, mandibular prognathism when older
- Hands are short and broad with a trident appearance, there is laxity of the ligaments
- Limbs show a rhizomelic (humerus/femur) shortening
- Examine spine for gibbus in infancy followed by lumbar lordosis and scoliosis in adolescence
- Examine cardiovascular system for evidence of pulmonary hypertension, secondary to recurrent sleep apnoea
- Offer to examine ears for chronic serous otitis media and teeth for dental malocclusion, which is common
- Offer to plot head circumference, height and weight on special achondroplasia charts (hydrocephalus can be an early complication), and to grade development

Your approach to the other chondrodysplastic syndromes (skeletal dysplasias) would be similar.

For example:

- Spondyloepiphyseal dysplasia
- Hypochondroplasia

Case – Child with spondyloepiphyseal dysplasia

I saw Julie. She is short but post pubertal. There is no obvious disproportion but she does look to have a skeletal dysplasia of some type with marked bony deformity including a marked kyphoscoliosis...

MUCOPOLYSACCHARIDOSES

Knowledge of the mucopolysaccharidoses and similar syndromes is important and a summary of the various conditions is listed. The candidate is referred to the further reading to read about the individual conditions in more detail.

Hurler's and Hunter's syndrome – coarse facial features obvious from the end of the bed.

Describe coarse facial features
- Thickened lips
- Large head with frontal bossing
- Flat midface
- Prominent sutures
- Broad flat nose

- Look at dorsum of wrist for carpal tunnel surgery correction scar (common)
- Examine corneas for clouding (appears after one year and not present in Hunter's)
- Examine fundi for cherry-red spot (present in GM-1 which is a differential)
- Comment on nasal discharge (common and persistent)
- Listen for upper airway obstruction
- Examine cardiovascular system for evidence of congestive cardiac failure
- Note umbilical hernia
- Examine for hepatosplenomegaly
- Note joint stiffness and contractures
- Examine spine for exaggerated kyphosis (usually present), gibbus, scoliosis and cervical rod surgery (common in Maroteaux-Lamy and Morquio)
- Offer to perform developmental examination, and expect it to be delayed

Difference between Hunter's and Hurler's

	Hunter's	Hurler's
Inheritance	X-linked *R*	~~AD~~ *AR*
Corneal clouding	no	yes
Severity	less	more
Nodules over scapulae	yes	no

DIFFERENTIAL DIAGNOSES

Other mucopolysaccharidoses

- Morquio – very severe physical features identical to Hurler's syndrome, but normal intelligence. Will have had cervical stabilisation surgery.
- Maroteaux-Lamy – phenotypically similar to Morquio's syndrome.
- Sanfilippo – less severe physical features, but profound mental retardation

Other differentials

- Multiple sulfatase deficiency (ichthyosis, more profound neurological deterioration)
- GM-1 gangliosidosis (pseudo-Hurler's)
- Mannosidosis (clinically like Hurler's without urinary findings)
- Fucosidosis (clinically like Hurler's without urinary findings)
- Mucolipidoses

SCHEME FOR EXAMINATION OF A CHILD WITH TALL STATURE

Tall children and adolescents are frequently seen in the exam.

INSTRUCTIONS

What do you think may be the cause of this child's tall stature?
Look at this child and describe what you see.

This is quite an open ended instruction and is best handled with a structure:

- Offer to plot child on height, weight and head circumference chart
- Ask parents' height. Is this a child with familial tall stature (see earlier).
- Is the child obviously dysmorphic? Marfan's syndrome, Klinefelter's syndrome, homocystinuria, Soto's syndrome (large head), Beckwith-Wiedemann syndrome (normal final height).
- Is there a goitre? Hyperthyroidism.

Marfan's syndrome

If the child looks Marfanoid move onto testing joint hyperextensibility, examine anterior chamber for lens dislocation, measure blood pressure, auscultate the heart and examine the palate. Remember that in Marfan's syndrome the lower segment of the body is longer than the upper segment and the arm span is greater than the height. Marfan's syndrome occurs 1:10,000 and is inherited as an autosomal dominant trait (defect in the fibrillin gene on chromosome 5). The diagnosis is a clinical one. Long term complications are aortic dissection/regurgitation, kyphoscoliosis and lens dislocation.

Marfan's commonly comes up in the exam and the clinical signs and management need to be thoroughly known.

It is essential to know the difference between Marfan's syndrome and homocystinuria.

	Marfan's	Homocystinuria
Joints	hyperextensible	contractures
Lens dislocation	up and in	down
Facies	long	ruddy complexion
Intelligence	normal	below average
Cardiac	aortic root dilation	normal
Bones	normal	osteoporosis
Urine	normal	excessive homocystine

Children with Marfan's syndrome will need yearly echocardiograms to compare their aortic root dimensions against centile charts, and regular ophthalmologic assessment. In the paediatric clinic it is important to monitor blood pressure regularly.

Case – Marfan's syndrome

Mark is a well looking boy who appears to be tall for his age, although I would like to plot him on a growth chart. He has a long thin face with dental crowding. He has arachnodactyly and hyper-extensible fingers. He can adduct his thumb across his palm (Sternberg's sign). His thumb and little finger overlap on encircling the opposite wrist. He has pectus excavatum. He can easily place the palms of his hands on to the floor with straight legs. His arm span appears to be greater than his height...

This would all be compatible with Marfan's syndrome. I would like to go on to examine his eyes and cardiovascular system...

OTHER CAUSES OF TALL STATURE

Klinefelter's syndrome (47XXY)

Individuals are tall with long limbs. It usually presents as delayed puberty with small testicles, rarely exceeding 2 ml volume. Gynaecomastia is present in 40% at puberty. Intelligence is below average and behavioural problems are common.

XYY syndrome

Children present with above average height and sub-normal intelligence. They have normal genitalia and pubertal development.

Soto's syndrome (cerebral gigantism)

Presents at birth as macrosomia and unusual facial features: prominent forehead and chin, large head circumference and hypertelorism. Hands, feet and genitalia can be large. Skeletal development is usually advanced so final adult height is usually normal.

TREATMENT OF TALL STATURE

This is rarely indicated. Aim is to reduce growth rate whilst accelerating bone maturation. Oestrogens are used in girls and reduce final height by 3–7 cm. Intervention in boys is with testosterone or somatostatin therapy.

YOUR NOTES

YOUR NOTES

CHAPTER 8 – DERMATOLOGY

Skin problems are commonly seen in the exam. Many skin lesions are part of systemic conditions such as Café-au-lait spots in neurofibromatosis and are covered elsewhere in the book. Specific skin conditions are discussed in this chapter. It is essential to know the appearance of the common skin lesions. The candidate is advised to revise the appearance of common skin lesions in a dermatology atlas (*see further reading*). This chapter has been written as notes on various aspects of skin conditions rather than case orientated for this reason.

SUMMARY

❑ Brief scheme for the examination of the skin
❑ Notes on skin examination
❑ Useful definitions
❑ Notes on specific conditions

BRIEF SCHEME FOR EXAMINATION OF THE SKIN

This is difficult and it is not possible to have a scheme which is always applicable
- Aim for good exposure
- Look at the hands, nails and mucous membranes
- Expose other areas
- If desperate ask if there is a rash and where it is
- Recognise common disorders

USEFUL NOTES ON SKIN EXAMINATION

Remember that examination of the skin includes a comment about the general appearance of the child, assessment of the skin, hair, nails and mucous membranes.

Describe the appearance of the skin in the appropriate language

1. Type of lesion: macule, papule, nodule, vesicle etc
2. Shape of individual lesions: round, oval, linear, annular etc
3. Distribution: (examine palms, soles, mouth, scalp)
4. Extent of involvement: circumscribed, regional, generalised
5. Pattern: symmetry, sun exposed area, sites of pressure etc
6. Characteristic location: flexural, extensor surface, palms and soles etc
7. Colour: red, brown, white etc. and whether blanches on pressure
8. Consistency of lesion: infiltrated, firm, soft, doughy etc

Look for lymphadenopathy, hepatosplenomegaly and at joints if appropriate.

Mention **Wood's lamp** examination for pigmented lesions.

Wood's lamp

This will highlight areas of altered pigmentation such as vitiligo and certain types of fungal infection. It is also used to look for the depigmented patches associated with tuberous sclerosis.

USEFUL DEFINITIONS

Macule: flat lesion that differs from surrounding because of its colour; may have any size, shape

Papule: small, solid, elevated (palpable) generally, 0.5 cm in diameter

Vesicle: circumscribed, elevated lesion containing clear fluid

Bullae: vesicle > 0.5 cm diameter

Weal: rounded, flat-topped papule or plaque that is evanescent, disappearing within hours

Plaque: elevation occupying large surface area formed by confluence of papules e.g. psoriasis

Nodule: palpable, solid, round or ellipsoid lesion larger than papule

Erosion: moist, circumscribed, depressed lesion due to loss of all or portion of viable epidermis

Pustule: circumscribed, raised lesion containing pus

Cyst: sac containing liquid, semi-solid material

Atrophy: diminution in the size of cell, tissue, organ or part of the body

Ulcer: defect in skin due to destruction of epidermis and part of dermis

Scar: ulcer heals with scar

Scale: abnormal shedding or accumulation of stratum corneum in flakes e.g. psoriasis

Crust: hardened deposits resulting from drying of exudate

Petechiae: pinpoint haemorrhage in the skin, does not blanch with pressure

Purpura: larger than petechiae, does not blanch with pressure

SKIN CONDITIONS COMMONLY SEEN IN THE EXAM

This list is not exhaustive but can be used as a revision checklist.

- Eczema
- Strawberry naevus
- Mongolian blue spot
- Psoriasis – (*see rheumatology chapter*)
- Capillary haemangioma (Sturge Weber) (*see neurology chapter*)
- Café-au-lait spots (Neurofibromatosis) (*see neurology chapter*)
- Sebaceous naevus
- Vitiligo
- Lipodystrophies
- Molluscum contagiosum
- Epidermolysis bullosa
- Ectodermal dysplasia

ECZEMA

- Chronic recurrent, genetically influenced skin disorder of early infancy, childhood and adult life
- Common problem – incidence 7:1000; prevalence 3–5% between 6 months and 10 years
- Associated with asthma/hay fever. Family history of atopy in 70%
- Slight female preponderance
- 70% cases begin < 2 years
- 65% have long term remission by 16 years
- Early onset, severe disease carries bad prognosis
- Distribution and morphology of lesion are diagnostic

Characteristic pattern of evolution

- Infantile phase begins between 1–6 months, lasts 2–3 years. Rash composed of red, itchy papules and plaques, many of which ooze and crust. Symmetrically distributed over the cheeks, forehead, scalp, trunk and extensor surfaces. Nappy area usually spared.
- Childhood phase between 4–10 years. Symmetrical distribution over wrists, ankles, flexural surfaces of arms, legs. Circumscribed, erythematous, scaly, lichenified plaques. May get secondarily infected.
- Adult phase mainly involves flexural creases of arms, legs, neck and hands/ feet
- Chronic pruritus leads to sleep loss, emotional upset
- Secondary infection with staphylococci, streptococci and herpes simplex require urgent treatment

Treatment

- Nail care, avoiding soap and biological detergents, avoid wool and rough clothing
- Emollients – emulsifying ointment, creams, bath oil
- Topical steroid preparations (the minimum potency to achieve the desired effect), wet wraps
- Antihistamines as antipruritic/sedative agent
- Allergen control – house dust mite
- Antibiotics for secondary infection

STRAWBERRY NAEVUS

Child aged 3 months with a prominent strawberry naevus on the upper abdomen (you should know what one looks like and therefore this should be easily identifiable).

QUESTIONS

What is it?
Will it get bigger?
Will it disappear?
What are the potential complications?

NOTES

- Common abnormality
- It is a capillary haemangioma, although this terminology is now seldom used (capillary refers to superficial and cavernous refers to deep)
- Bright red, protuberant, compressible, sharply demarcated
- Usually not present at birth but appears within 2 months
- More common in females than males
- Common sites – face, scalp, back, anterior chest – may be multiple
- Develops in phases – rapid expansion (during first year), stationary (6–12 months) and spontaneous involution (develops blanched, pale, grey areas)
- 60% involute by 5 years, 90% by 9 years
- Involution does not correlate with size or site of lesion except for lip lesions which usually persist
- In general no treatment is required and the parents are reassured in view of good outcome
- Complications – ulceration, infection, haemorrhage, platelet consumption. May interfere with vision (interfering with the development of binocular vision), urination (urethra), airway (tracheo-bronchial).
- Treatment is sometimes needed for very large lesions or lesions in which complications have arisen – options include excision, laser (much better when used for flat capillary haemangioma), corticosteroid/interferon.

MONGOLIAN BLUE SPOT

This is a reasonably common short case. You may be asked to look at purplish pigmentation over the lower back of a baby. The differential (a real one in clinical practice) is bruising and the possibility of non-accidental injury may be raised.

- Bluish-black macules over lumbosacral area and buttocks of most negro and oriental babies
- Collection of melanocytes in dermis
- Mistaken for bruising/NAI
- Fade gradually
- No clinical significance

SEBACEOUS NAEVUS

This case would present as a spot diagnosis and like the other common skin conditions it is well worth looking up the appearance in a book.

- Solitary, oval or linear, yellow-orange, warty lesion on the scalp
- Circumscribed area of hair loss
- Treatment – surgical excision
- Risk of neoplastic change (basal cell carcinoma) in 10–15% cases after puberty

LIPODYSTROPHY

Lipodystrophy is a loss of subcutaneous fat. You may see a child with either generalised or partial lipodystrophy. The clue is the prominent muscles with reduced subcutaneous fat particularly over the face. It is important to have some knowledge of the causes and types of lipodystrophy.

Generalised lipodystrophy

- Congenital (autosomal recessive) or acquired (sporadic)
- Tall children, advanced skeletal maturation, prominent muscles, enlargement of penis/clitoris, abundant curly scalp hair
- Acanthosis nigricans, hirsutism, hepatomegaly, insulin-resistant diabetes
- May have renal, cardiac, neurological abnormality, seizures, developmental delay, carbohydrate intolerance, hyperinsulinaemia, hypertriglyceridaemia
- Growth hormone low despite tall stature

Partial lipodystrophy

- F>M (4:1)
- Develops over few months to several years
- Symmetrical subcutaneous fat loss initially over the face, upper trunks and arms – leads to disproportion between the upper and lower limbs
- Chronic glomerulonephritis associated in 25% cases with low C3 complement due to activation of alternate pathway
- No treatment, prognosis is guarded

Diabetes

Lipoatrophy and lipohypertrophy can occur at injection sites.

VITILIGO

- Symmetrical, ivory-white de-pigmented patches
- Common problem; higher incidence in pigmented population. 50% present under 20 years of age
- Associated with autoimmune diseases (thyroid, diabetes, pernicious anaemia, Addison's disease)
- Slow progression, static after variable period of time
- Spontaneous re-pigmentation uncommon 10–20% cases
- Caucasians usually require only camouflage make-up

MOLLUSCUM CONTAGIOSUM

- Smooth, pearly papules with characteristic central punctum
- Caused by pox virus
- Occurs in crops, spreads by auto-inoculation
- Mostly no treatment is offered and the condition improves over 12–18 months
- Cryotherapy with liquid nitrogen and curettage has been used

PSORIASIS

- Common disorder, prevalence 1–3%; 20% develop rash < 20 years. Characterised by red, well-demarcated plaques with a dry, thick, silvery scale.
- Multi-factorial – both hereditary and environmental factors involved
- Family history in 1/3rd cases
- Distribution: scalp, sacrum, and extensor surfaces of extremities. 50% children have large plaques over knees, elbows.
- Guttate psoriasis – drop-like lesions scattered all over body including face, trunk, extremities in 1/3rd cases.
- Persistent nappy area dermatitis in infancy
- Other variants – erythrodermic and pustular psoriasis
- Arthritis seen in 10% cases
- Koebner phenomenon – lesions induced in areas of local injury
- Auspitz sign – removal of scale causes multiple, small bleeding points
- Diagnosis clinical, can be confirmed on skin biopsy
- Course chronic and unpredictable
- Treatment – tar, keratolytics, corticosteroids.
- Chronic lesions may require PUVA regime with psoralen and UV light.

ICHTHYOSIS

Ichthyosis implies dry and thick skin of varying severity. It is separate from eczema in which inflammatory change plays a key role. There are various specific syndromes.

- Group of inherited conditions with dry, thickened skin of varying severity

Types
- Ichthyosis vulgaris – autosomal dominant
- Lameller ichthyosis – autosomal recessive
- Congenital ichthyosiform erythroderma (CIE) – autosomal recessive
- Bullous – autosomal dominant

- Lifelong disorder, little spontaneous remission
- Typical histopathology
- Presents at birth 'collodion baby' (lamellar and ichthyosiform erythroderma) and within 3 months in other types
- Collodion baby encased at birth in shiny, tight membrane
- Thick scales, corneal dystrophy, ectropion, fever and failure to thrive
- Treatment: emollients, keratolytics, oral retinoids (CIE), antibiotics for secondary infection
- Associated syndromes – Netherton, chondrodysplasia punctata

ECTODERMAL DYSPLASIA

INSTRUCTION

Comment on this child's general appearance

> **Case**
>
> *Simon is a well looking child with coarse wispy hair and sparse eyebrows and eyelashes. His skin appears to be dry. He has peri-orbital hyperpigmentation. He has pegged teeth (or false teeth)*

This would fit in with anhidrotic ectodermal dysplasia

NOTES ON ECTODERMAL DYSPLASIA

- Heterogeneous group of inherited conditions with primary defect in one or more of teeth, nails, hair, sweat gland function and other ectodermal tissue e.g. eyes, ears, oral/nasal mucosa, melanocytes and central nervous system
- Diverse features
- Scalp hair very sparse, wig is useful
- Reduced number of conical teeth, need for early use of prostheses
- Nails – thick, dystrophic and fragile
- Hypohydrosis leads to life threatening hyperthermia; advice on cooling, activity, clothing, relocation to cooler areas important
- Skin – atrophic, dry, wrinkled; require emollients
- Eye – dry eyes, hypoplasia of nasolacrimal duct may lead to corneal ulcers
- Facies – thick lips, saddle nose, frontal bossing, maxillary hypoplasia, abnormal ears
- Mucosa – dry mouth, thick nasal secretions, atrophic rhinitis, recurrent chest infections, dysphagia, urethral stones and carcinomas
- Inheritance: X-linked recessive/autosomal recessive/autosomal dominant
- Asthma may be associated
- Regular follow up indicated for mucosal leukoplakia and blood dyscrasia

Management

- Precautions – protection from exposure to high ambient temperatures
- Early dental treatment
- Artificial tears
- Wig

EPIDERMOLYSIS BULLOSA

- Mixed group of hereditary, bullous diseases characterised by the development, in response to trauma, of vesicles, bullae or erosions
- Over 15 types based on inheritance, clinical features, electron microscopic identification of cleavage plane of blister – epidermolytic (within epidermis), junctional (at the dermoepidermal junction in the lamina lucida) or dermatolytic (upper dermis)
- Autosomal dominant form of non-scarring epidermolysis bullosa simplex (EBS) is present at birth, mucous membrane may be involved. Feet and hand lesions are common but may be generalised. Usually improves with time.
- Localised type of EBS – confined to hands/feet. Usually in first 2 years of life. May be confused with friction blister (autosomal dominant).
- Junctional EB – autosomal recessive, present at birth or shortly thereafter, often progressive. Death is common. Nails are lost, teeth are dysplastic. Large granulomatous ulcers seen in perioral area. Mucosal involvement may lead to oesophageal strictures. Anaemia, secondary infection common complication.
- Dystrophic EB – autosomal recessive, most severe with devastating effects. Usually present at birth. Entire skin may be affected by minor trauma. Scarring, milia formation and nail loss occur. Oral involvement with scarring of tongue and oesophageal stricture seen. Mitten-like hands/feet, contracture of large joints often result. Poor prognosis. Complications: infection, anaemia, growth retardation, amyloidosis, skin cancer etc.
- Management: supportive – nutrition, transfusion, gentle handling to minimise trauma, dressing of lesions, antibiotics for infection, appropriate clothing and footwear. Multidisciplinary involvement.

YOUR NOTES

YOUR NOTES

YOUR NOTES

CHAPTER 9 – RHEUMATOLOGY

The examination of joints can come up as part of the examination of another system or as a short case in its own right. It is an opportunity with good knowledge of joint examination and abnormal pathology to score well. It is essential to practise joint examination carefully and frequently and to recognise and understand the range of normality. We have been quite thorough including some of this information under the notes on specific joints. We have also listed some of the scenarios which you may come across in the exam.

SUMMARY
❑ Approach to joint examination
❑ Notes on specific joints
❑ Neonatal hip examination
❑ Examination of the hands
❑ Juvenile chronic arthritis
❑ Psoriatic arthritis
❑ Dermatomyositis
❑ Haemophilia
❑ Osteogenesis imperfecta
❑ Hemihypertrophy
❑ Nerve injuries
❑ Short neck
❑ Plagiocephaly
❑ Toe walking
❑ Foot drop
❑ Orthoses
❑ Talipes
❑ Perthes' disease

APPROACH TO JOINT EXAMINATION

Always take a general look at the child first

Bear in mind the symptoms of joint disease

Symptoms

- Pain
- Stiffness
- Swelling
- Instability
- Locking
- Clicking
- Loss of function

Examination involves following components

- **LOOK**
- **FEEL**
- **MOVE**
- **ASSESS FUNCTION**

General

The following is a guide only. All aspects of joint examination do not necessarily need to be carried out in every short case. If there is an obvious abnormality e.g. swollen left knee or swollen interphalangeal joints then this needs to be focused on.

Look

General appearance of the child. Any obvious clues e.g. orthoses, shoes, splints.

Look for any deformity, erythema, swelling around the joint, scars from previous infection or surgery and muscle. Compare with normal joint.

Feel

Watch patient's face while palpating the joint. Feel for skin temperature, tenderness, and joint effusion.

Move

Ask the child to move the joint before you move it to ensure that movement is not painful and to get some idea of the range of movement possible. It is important to do this as you don't want to cause pain as soon as you touch the patient!

Function

Make the patient stand up and walk a short distance (gait) with exposure. Similarly for upper limbs, get the patient to do things which he/she finds difficult e.g. drinking from cup, grasping large objects like bottle/box and small objects like paper clips etc. Make him/her write, draw, comb hair, take off shirt etc.

If the affected joint is not obvious the order for examination may be from hand to head, and head to toe, i.e. hands, wrists, elbows, shoulders, temporo-mandibular joints, spine, hips, knees, ankles, feet.

NOTES ON SPECIFIC JOINTS

Hands and wrists

Described under examination of hand (see later).

Elbows

Range of movement – flexion 135°, extension 0°, supination 90°, and pronation 90°. Supination and pronation are tested with elbows flexed.

Shoulders

Range of movement can be tested easily:

- 'Put your hands above your head'; tests flexion (90°), and abduction (180°)
- 'Give yourself a hug'; tests adduction (45°)
- 'Scratch your back'; tests external rotation (45°)
- 'Hide your hands behind your back'; tests internal rotation (55°) and extension (45°)

Jaw and cervical spine

Movement at temporo-mandibular joint should be examined with the child opening and closing mouth. Feel for crepitus over temporo-mandibular joint and look for acquired micrognathia and dental malocclusion. Range of movement at cervical spine is – flexion (45°), extension (50°), rotation (80°) and lateral flexion (40°).

Thoracolumbar spine

Examine child standing and bending forward for kyphoscoliosis. Feel for tenderness and check range of movement; flexion (should be able to touch toes), extension (30° at lumbar area), lateral bending (50° to each side), lateral rotation (30° to each side). Functional evaluation – ask the child to pick an object up from floor or put socks and shoes on.

Lower limbs

Examine the gait; make the child squat (for proximal muscle weakness) and stand on each leg (for Trendelenburg's sign). The examination of gait is covered in detail in the neurology chapter.

Hips

Look for muscle wasting and note the resting position. Feel for tenderness. Measure true leg length between anterior superior iliac spine and medial malleolus. Range of movement – flexion (120°), extension (30°), internal rotation (35°), external rotation (45°), abduction (50°) and adduction (30°). Stabilise the pelvis before checking the range of movement.

Knees

Look for quadriceps wasting and feel for tenderness, raised local temperature and effusion. Check range of movement: flexion (135°), extension (up to 10°). Check for abnormal movement.

Ankles and feet

Range of movement at ankle: plantar flexion (50°), dorsiflexion (20°). Inversion (5°) and eversion (5°) occurs at sub-talar joint. Abduction (10°) and adduction (20°) occurs at mid-tarsal joints. First metatarso-phalyngeal joint permits plantar flexion (45°) and extension (70°).

TRENDELENBURG GAIT

Non-painful limp

Trendelenburg positive implies the affected hip is lower than the unaffected hip e.g. hip dislocation, instability or muscle weakness.

Painful limp

Trendelenburg negative implies the affected hip is higher than the unaffected hip e.g. Perthes' disease.

EXTRA-ARTICULAR MANIFESTATIONS

It may be relevant to extend your examination to look for extra-articular manifestations of joint disease.

e.g. Skin – psoriasis
     Eyes – juvenile chronic arthritis

This is covered under specific cases – see later.

NEONATAL HIP EXAMINATION

There is a 'hip' doll available and often used in the exam. There is therefore a need to know precisely the correct methods of hip examination, the potential abnormalities and how they are dealt with. You may also be asked about the role of ultrasound in the detection of hip problems in the neonatal period.

Barlow test

Stabilise the pelvis with one hand by lying the child on its back with its hips flexed and knees bent. Place the middle finger of each hand over the greater trochanter and the thumb on the inside of the thigh opposite the lesser trochanter. Push down on the hip, creating a posterior force, and you should feel the hip dislocate if abnormal.

Ortolani test

This is the test to relocate the recently dislocated hip. The hips are flexed and abducted and the femoral head should move back into the acetabulum.

In practice, these two tests are performed together in one movement.

NOTES ON ABNORMALITIES DETECTED ON NEONATAL HIP EXAMINATION

The abnormalities detected fall into different groups:

- Dislocated
- Dislocatable
- Unstable/click

The first two groups require urgent orthopaedic input and splinting – double nappies or Pavlik harness. The latter group require further assessment and follow up and many in this group improve with time.

It would be sensible to discuss with your local orthopaedic surgeons their strategy for the management of hip problems in the neonatal period. In some units ultrasound is offered either to all babies or to families with risk factors. Other hospitals do not offer this and there is no consensus as yet.

EXAMINATION OF THE HANDS

This is very important and is the starting point of the clinical examination of most systems. Alternatively, you may be asked just to look at the hands. In most cases the features are obvious and lead you on to further examination. In other circumstances a more detailed review of potential pathology in the hand is required and the following is a suggested scheme.

Hand = important part of clinical examination.

INSTRUCTION
Examine this child's hands

EXAMINATION
Static examination

- General inspection – shape, size, colour, temperature, sweating, swelling, scars (venepuncture – preterm)
- Individual tissues – skin, nails, fat and fascia, blood vessels, nerve, muscle, tendon, tendon sheath, joint, bones

Function – more information gained from observing the functional use of hand.

General inspection

Look first for any obvious abnormality which if found will determine the rest of your examination. If there is no obvious lead then work through the sequence below.

- Obvious swelling or deformity
- Abnormality of the skin or nails
- Scars – preterm venepuncture

Movement – spontaneous, gestures, tremors

Posture

- 'Claw hand' – hyperextension of metacarpophalangeal joint and lack of extension of interphalangeal joint due to weakness of interossei (damage to medial cord of brachial plexus at birth)
- Hemiplegia – flexed hand and arm
- Wrist drop – radial palsy
- Ulnar deviation – rheumatoid arthritis

Shape

- Trauma
- Arachnodactyly – Marfan's syndrome
- Pseudohypoparathyroidism – short 4th, 5th metacarpal

Size

- Broad hands, stubby fingers, curved little finger, simian crease – Down's syndrome
- Large – acromegaly (rare)

Colour, temperature, sweating

Detailed features (individual tissues)
- Skin – eczema, contact dermatitis, scleroderma
- Nails – clubbing (respiratory system), psoriasis – pitting of nails, onycholysis and arthropathy of distal interphalangeal joint, koilonychia – iron deficiency anaemia, splinter haemorrhage, white bands (horizontal) – abnormal zones of nail growth in serious illness, malnutrition, and chemotherapy.
- Subcutaneous fat and palmer fascia – Dupuytren's contracture (rare in childhood) – indicative of chronic liver disease.
- Blood vessels – nail bed telangiectasia in dermatomyositis, haemorrhage in nail fold in vasculitis e.g. dermatomyositis, rheumatoid arthritis and scleroderma. Raynaud's phenomenon in primary Raynaud's disease.
- Tendon sheaths – in rheumatoid arthritis thickening of synovial sheath leads to swelling on the dorsum of wrist, front of finger and wrist.

- Joints – arthritis can cause anything from mild spindling of proximal interphalangeal joints to gross disorganisation of hand with subluxation of joints and wasting of small muscles. Psoriatic arthritis involves the distal interphalangeal joints and nails.
- Bones – may show fracture, bony prominence, congenital abnormalities.

Function

- Function of hand is best assessed by simple tests like grip strength, use of spoon, knife and fork, holding cup, drawing with pencil, writing, doing and undoing buttons etc.
- Range of movement at metacarpophalangeal joint – flexion 90°, extension 30°. Proximal interphalangeal joint – flexion 100°
- Distal interphalangeal joint – flexion 90°, extension 10°

Wrist

- Wrist is held in flexion with pronation of forearm in cerebral palsy. Diffuse swelling of wrist may be seen in arthritis. Palpate to localise tenderness.
- Range of movements – flexion 80°, extension 70°, radial deviation 20°, ulnar deviation 30°

Elbows

See earlier – worth a look if psoriasis is suspected based on the appearance of the nails

JUVENILE CHRONIC ARTHRITIS

This is a very common case. Most patients attend outpatients and physiotherapy only and are rarely seen on the wards. The use of methotrexate has revolutionised the management of chronic arthritis. This means children seen may have very few physical signs.

INSTRUCTION

Please examine Bethany's hands. She is 10 years old.

> *Introduce yourself. I would like to plot her height and weight on the centile chart. Bethany has got bilateral swollen wrists. There is painful restriction of range of movement at both wrists to around 120°. I can also see marked swelling of proximal interphalangeal joints of index and middle fingers bilaterally. I would like to do a detailed examination of all joints...proceed.*

This scenario gives you a good opportunity to say what else you would examine.

For example

- I would like to examine for signs of eye disease (*see later*)
- I would like to review the growth
- I would look for signs of steroid toxicity (*see renal chapter*)
- I would like to check the skin

NOTES ON JUVENILE CHRONIC ARTHRITIS

These notes are quite thorough. A good knowledge of this potentially confusing area is essential.

Prevalence

65:100,000 schoolchildren.

Criteria for classification

- Age of onset < 16 years
- Arthritis in one or more joints defined as swelling or effusion, or presence of two or more of the following signs: limitation of range of motion, tenderness or pain on movement, and increased heat
- Duration of disease minimum 3 months

Polyarticular: 5 or more joints
Pauciarticular: 4 or fewer joints
Systemic disease: arthritis with intermittent fever

Systemic onset juvenile chronic arthritis

20% of juvenile chronic arthritis. Onset throughout childhood. Equal sex incidence. Systemic symptoms: fever, macular, non-pruritic rash; polyarticular arthritis. Other features: lymphadenopathy, hepato-splenomegaly, pericarditis, anaemia, leucocytosis, and thrombocytosis. Systemic features may precede arthritis by months. Rheumatoid factor (RF) and antinuclear antibody (ANA) negative. No eye involvement or sacroiliitis. Progress to severe and long term arthritis in 25% cases.

Pauciarticular juvenile chronic arthritis type 1 (early onset)

35–40% of juvenile chronic arthritis. Onset during early childhood (2–5 years). 80% girls. Few large joints: knee, ankle, elbow. Chronic uveitis occurs in 30%, often asymptomatic, can cause blindness. ANA positivity (90%) correlates with the risk of uveitis. No sacroiliitis; HLA DR5, DRW6, DRW8. Prognosis is excellent except for eyesight (ocular damage 10%), polyarthritis develops eventually in 20% cases.

Pauciarticular juvenile chronic arthritis type 2 (late onset)

10–15% of juvenile chronic arthritis. 90% boys. Onset during late childhood. Few large joints especially hip girdle involved; sacroiliitis common. Acute uveitis in 10–20% cases. ANA and RF negative. HLA B27 positive in 75% cases. Many develop ankylosing spondylitis.

Polyarticular rheumatoid factor negative juvenile chronic arthritis

20–25% of juvenile chronic arthritis. 90% girls. Onset at any age. Symmetrical arthritis involving both large and small joints of upper and lower limbs but no sacroiliitis. Uveitis is rare. RF negative, ANA positive in 25% cases. Prognosis: severe arthritis in 10–15% cases.

Polyarticular rheumatoid factor positive juvenile chronic arthritis

5–10% of juvenile chronic arthritis. 80% girls. Late childhood. Resembles adult rheumatoid arthritis with symmetric polyarthritis affecting upper and lower limbs. RF positive 100%; ANA 75%. HLA DR4. No uveitis, sacroiliitis rare. Prognosis: severe erosive arthritis with poor functional outcome in 50% cases.

Eye problems in juvenile chronic arthritis

All anti-nuclear antibody positive patients are at risk of uveitis and hence need regular slit-lamp examination by ophthalmologist. Active disease is treated with steroid eye drops and mydriatics. Chronic uveitis can progress to poor vision with a cloudy cornea and fixed constricted pupil.

NOTES ON MANAGEMENT OF JUVENILE CHRONIC ARTHRITIS

Summary

This question is commonly asked and it is very important to give a summary answer at the outset with appropriate emphasis. This is a good opportunity to show the examiner that you appreciate the multi-disciplinary management of a complex and chronic condition like juvenile chronic arthritis.

Management of juvenile chronic arthritis	
Physiotherapy and occupational therapy	hydrotherapy passive movement splints
Medical therapy	non-steroidal anti-inflammatory drugs local or systemic steroids disease modifying drugs e.g. methotrexate

Drugs

1. Non-steroidal anti-inflammatory drugs remain the first line particularly ibuprofen. Doses are usually high and antacids are occasionally required for gastrointestinal side-effects.
2. Corticosteroid injection (triamcinolone) – useful in oligo-articular disease. They are increasingly used early in severely inflamed joints with good results. Systemic corticosteroids in severe disease – particularly disease with systemic manifestations.
3. Disease modifying drugs like methotrexate

Non-drug treatment

This is very important and in the exam it is essential that you transmit to the examiner your awareness of non-medical therapies.

Physiotherapy and occupational therapy

- Hydrotherapy
- Passive movement
- Gentle exercises
- Splints

PSORIATIC ARTHRITIS

INSTRUCTION

Could you examine John's hands. He is 12 years old.

> *Introduce yourself. John is 12 years old. I would like to plot his weight and height on a centile chart. Examination of his hands shows diffusely swollen right index finger at the distal interphalangeal joint. On closer examination, I can clearly see multiple pits on the nail of this finger. I would like to carry out further joint examination and look for the rash of psoriasis...proceed.*

What else would you like to examine?

- Joint examination – asymmetric oligoarthritis of large and small joints
- Rash – typical of psoriasis. Erythematous papules which coalesce to form plaques with silvery or yellow-white scales. Preferred sites are scalp, knees, elbows, umbilicus and genitalia
- Nails may show multiple pits, vertical or horizontal ridging; onycholysis is uncommon
- Eye examination may show chronic uveitis similar to juvenile chronic arthritis

NOTES ON PSORIATIC ARTHRITIS

Chronic inflammatory arthritis before 16 years of age, preceded by, accompanied by, or followed within 15 years by psoriasis. Prevalence is expected to be from 10–15 cases per 100,000. Age at onset usually around 10 years. F>M 1.2:1.

Vancouver criteria for diagnosis

Definite psoriatic arthritis

> Arthritis with typical psoriatic rash
> Arthritis with three of the four following minor criteria
>> Dactylitis
>> Nail pitting or onycholysis
>> Psoriasis like rash
>> Family history (1st or 2nd degree relatives) of psoriasis

Probable psoriatic arthritis

> Arthritis with 2 of the 4 minor criteria

Psoriatic arthritis should be suspected in chronic arthritis with dactylitis or asymmetric involvement of large or small joints, particularly the first metatarsophalangeal or the distal interphalangeal joints. The diagnosis is clinical. Rheumatoid factor is absent. ANA may be seen in 17–50% cases. Management is on the same lines as juvenile chronic arthritis. Many children with pauciarticular disease may progress to polyarticular disease, some requiring major reconstructive surgery of hips and other joints. Course may be relapsing and remitting with or without flaring of skin disease.

JUVENILE DERMATOMYOSITIS

This is an unusual case and a rare condition in clinical practice. The following will help to increase your awareness of the condition and will be of practical use if you see a case.

INSTRUCTION

Would you examine Jamie who is 6 years old with a rash over his eyelids?

> *I would like to plot his height and weight on the centile chart. He has got a purplish macular rash over both upper eyelids also extending partly over the nasal bridge. I can also see papular rash over his knuckles on both sides. I would like to examine him for proximal muscle weakness...*

What else would you like to examine?

Dermatomyositis

- 20% present in childhood, usually the second decade
- Acute or sub-acute onset
- Painful tender muscles with lethargy, skin rashes and proximal muscle weakness either shoulder girdle or lower limbs
- Usually asymmetrical
- Rash – characteristic – upper eyelids and upper cheeks (butterfly), rash also over elbows, hyperaemia of nail beds
- Can get dysphagia (adults), skin calcification
- Raised ESR and CPK
- Confirm diagnosis with muscle biopsy
- Treatment difficult and with long term steroids +/- other immunosuppression

HAEMOPHILIA
INSTRUCTION
Examine this young man's elbow

> *Introduce yourself. On inspection, there is no obvious swelling or redness. On feeling the joint, there is no tenderness. On both passive and active movement there is a fixed flexion deformity of the elbow, although the joint is not painful. I note there is also some bruising to the upper arm.*

This would be compatible with haemophilia.

Supplementary questions
- How does arthropathy reflect the seriousness of the haemophilia?
- How do you treat bleeding into the joint?

NOTES ON HAEMOPHILIA

The haemophilia's are the commonest and the most serious of the congenital coagulation disorders. About 80% of cases are the X-linked haemophilia A, causing a majority to have reduced factor VIII activity and factor VIII antigen. Numerous mutations in gene structure have been described. In 80% of cases the family history is positive. The severity of disease depends on the level of factor VIII activity in the plasma – severe cases have <1% of normal activity, moderate cases have 1–5%, and mild cases have 6–30%. The commonest time of presentation is when ambulation begins. The hallmark is haemarthroses; knees, ankles and elbows being the most commonly affected joints. The bleeding itself occurs from the vascular synovium. Repeated haemorrhages may cause degenerative changes with osteoporosis, muscle atrophy and eventually a fixed immobile joint.

The factor VIII deficiency causes a greatly prolonged partial thromboplastin time, with a normal platelet count, bleeding time and prothrombin time.

Management of haemophilia and other bleeding disorders, requires multidisciplinary expertise, mostly in haemophilia centres. The mainstay of medical treatment, for those with severe haemophilia, is the administration of factor VIII concentrates. These can be given in two ways: either as prophylaxis against haemorrhage or as required for acute bleeding. Mild to moderate haemophiliacs often only require the administration of DDAVP. Prenatal diagnosis is now possible. The gene is known and there is a gene probe.

The problems with factor VIII replacement therapy fall into two main groups:

1. Blood borne diseases, particularly HIV, hepatitis D and hepatitis C – this has been helped by the development of recombinant factor VIII concentrate which is in use but expensive.
2. The development of factor VIII inhibitors, which render factor VIII replacement therapy ineffective through antibody neutralisation and require progressively higher doses to be given.

OSTEOGENESIS IMPERFECTA

INSTRUCTION

Examine Clara's eyes please

Introduce yourself. The most obvious feature is the blue sclera.

With that in mind, what would you like to examine?

I would like to go on and look for bony deformities in the arms and legs, with the diagnosis of osteogenesis imperfecta in mind.

Mum may be in a wheelchair in which case that is an obvious clue

This is a very common short case. The main clues being the blue sclera and the presence of the mother in a wheelchair reflecting the autosomal dominant inheritance of the condition.

Supplementary questions

- What different types of osteogenesis imperfecta are there?
- What is the inheritance?
- What is the differential (NAI)?
- What do you see in the skull of the newborn? - wormian bones

NOTES ON OSTEOGENESIS IMPERFECTA

Osteogenesis imperfecta is a disorder of connective tissue characterised by bone fragility. The disease encompasses a phenotypically and genetically heterogeneous group of inherited disorders that result from mutations in the genes that encode for type 1 collagen. The disorder is manifest in the tissues in which the principal matrix is collagen, namely bone, sclerae and ligaments. The musculoskeletal manifestations vary from perinatal lethal forms, to moderate forms with deformity and a propensity to fracture, to clinically silent forms with subtle osteopenia and no deformity, as overleaf:

Osteogenesis imperfecta type I

This is characterised by osteoporosis and excessive bone fragility, distinctly blue sclera and hearing loss. Autosomal dominant inheritance, 1 in 30,000 live births. Fractures may be obvious from birth. Hearing impairment due to otosclerosis affects most patients by the 5th decade, but is rare in the 1st decade. Some families have dentinogenesis imperfecta – with yellow transparent teeth which are fragile. There is spontaneous improvement with puberty. X-rays show generalised osteopenia, evidence of previous fractures and callus formation at the site of new bone formation. The skull X-ray shows wormian bones.

Osteogenesis imperfecta type II

This lethal syndrome characterised by low birth weight and typical X-ray findings of crumpled bones and beaded ribs. Autosomal recessive in a few cases, most being autosomal dominant new mutations. Affect 1 in 60,000 live births. 50% are stillborn, the remainder dying soon after birth from respiratory difficulty due to a defective thoracic cage. It is worth looking at a picture of the lethal form. X-rays show multiple fracture of the ribs, often beaded, and crumpled (accordion like) appearance of the long bones.

Osteogenesis imperfecta type III

This syndrome is characterised by severe bone fragility and multiple fractures in the newborn period which lead to progressive skeletal deformity. The sclera may be bluish at birth, but become less blue with age. Autosomal recessive with clinical variability suggesting genetic heterogeneity. Few patients survive into adult life. X-rays show generalised osteopenia and multiple fractures, without the beading or crumpling of the ribs seen in type II.

Osteogenesis imperfecta type IV

This syndrome is characterised by osteoporosis leading to bone fragility without the other features of type I. The sclera may be bluish at birth, but become less blue as the patient matures. Autosomal dominant inheritance. Variable age of onset and variable number of fractures, there is spontaneous improvement with puberty. X-rays show generalised osteopenia, and fractures, but these are generally less than the other forms of osteogenesis imperfecta.

Management

For osteogenesis imperfecta type II, no therapeutic intervention is helpful. For other forms, careful nursing of the newborn may prevent excessive fractures. Beyond the newborn period, aggressive orthopaedic treatment is the mainstay of treatment aimed at prompt splinting of fractures and correction of deformities. Genetic counselling is important. Reliable prenatal diagnosis is not available for all forms of osteogenesis imperfecta, although severely affected foetuses may be confidently recognised by X-rays, USS and biochemistry.

HEMIHYPERTROPHY

This is often difficult to recognise. It may involve the whole of one side of the body, or be limited in extent e.g. to just one leg. It may be congenital, in which case the tissues are structurally and functionally normal. It has been associated with mental retardation, ipsilateral paired internal organs and rarely with Wilms' tumours or adrenal carcinomas. Hemihypertrophy can be confused with regional overgrowth secondary to neurofibromatosis type I, haemangiomas and lymphangiomas.

Hemihypertrophy occurs in 25% of Beckwith-Weidemann syndrome (see page 108)

NERVE INJURIES

Nerve injuries are common. They make good spot cases and should be revised carefully.

INSTRUCTION

Examine Steven's hands. He is 10 years old.

> *Steven looks well. Looking at his hands, there is atrophy of thenar muscles and loss of thenar eminence in the right hand. Hypothenar muscles are well preserved. I would like to do full motor examination of both upper limbs...continue.*

Diagnosis – median nerve palsy

Examine also for:

- Muscle wasting of arms, forearms
- Classic signs of brachial plexus lesions: 'claw hand' in Klumpke's palsy; 'waiter's tip' hand in Erb's palsy
- Classic signs of peripheral nerve lesion: wrist drop in radial nerve palsy; 'monkey hand' in median nerve palsy; and 'claw hand' in ulnar nerve palsy.
- Fasciculation indicative of anterior horn cell disease
- Contractures
- Scars in the hand, neck and the back
- Scoliosis

NOTES ON PERIPHERAL NERVE PALSIES

Ulnar nerve palsy

- Sensory loss medial 1½ fingers
- Motor claw hand, weakness and wasting of small muscles with sparing of thenar eminence

Median nerve palsy

- Sensory loss of thumb and lateral 2½ fingers with wasting of thenar eminence.
- Motor weakness of thenar eminence, opponens pollicis, lateral two lumbricals, adductor pollicis brevis

Radial nerve palsy

- Sensory loss in anatomical snuffbox
- Motor loss wrist, finger and thumb extension weakness of extensors of wrist, thumb, MCP joints of fingers, 'wrist drop'

Erb's palsy

C5,6, R>L, can be bilateral. Occurs secondary to difficult deliveries, particularly shoulder dystocia. Usually reflects compression with haemorrhage and oedema and there is a good recovery. Occasionally the nerve is torn.

Features

- Asymmetric Moro
- Adduction and internal rotation at the shoulder
- Extension at the elbow
- Pronation of the forearm
- Flexion of the wrist (waiter's tip)
- Limb is hypotonic with a reduce biceps jerk

Associations

- Fractured clavicle
- Horner's syndrome

Management

- Physiotherapy
- Surgery (rarely)

Klumpke's

- Much less common = claw hand (C8,T1)

MISCELLANEOUS NOTES

Short neck

There are different causes of a short neck and you may come across a child in the exam with a short neck and need to be aware of the differential diagnosis.

- Turner's syndrome
- Skeletal dysplasia
- Klippel-Feil syndrome

Plagiocephaly

This is increasingly common as a phenomenon. Most plagiocephaly is simple, does not imply a craniosynostoses and improves with follow up.

In a child, for example with a prominent left occiput who is growing and developing normally one would not consider surgery.

It is essential however to be aware of some of the more common craniosynostoses and the relevant syndromes including Crouzon's and Apert's and the candidate is advised to go through this subject in one of the larger paediatric texts (See Further Reading, page 294).

Toe walking

- Can be a normal finding up until age 3
- Neurological disorders include cerebral palsy, Duchenne muscular dystrophy, spinal cord problems, congenital tendo-achilles shortening
- Leg length discrepancy
- Habit

Foot drop

- Variety of causes
- Patient has a stepping gait and lifts the affected limb high to avoid scraping the foot on the floor. They are unable to walk on their heel.
- Possible causes   – lateral popliteal nerve palsy (look for signs of injury below and lateral to the affected knee)
  - peroneal muscle atrophy
  - poliomyelitis

Orthoses

- Children with neurological disorders are very prone to developing joint contractures and bony abnormalities, particularly spinal kyphoscoliosis
- Orthoses are useful in helping to prevent contractures, in maintaining a good position if contractures have been repaired and in providing joint stability
- They are particularly useful in aiding individual children with mobility
- The type of orthoses depends on the child's individual needs e.g. they may be ankle foot orthoses if there is just ankle and foot involvement, extending to the knee if the knee is involved
- Should there be a scoliosis, thoracolumbar orthoses are available

Talipes

2 types – positional and non-positional

- Positional talipes occurs due to the in-utero position, and requires, at most, some parental physiotherapy
- Non-positional talipes or clubfoot is a multifactorial deformity of primarily genetic origin, 30–50% require casting only to recover, the cast being applied within the first week. The casts are changed weekly. Surgery is reserved for those not responding to casting. If surgery is required, usually at 6–9 months, it involves lengthening the tight tendons and releasing tight joints with pinning and casting – usually with good results. 3% recurrence risk in future children.

Perthes' disease

- Differential diagnosis of limp
- Arises from disturbance of the upper femoral epiphysis secondary to ischaemic necrosis of unknown aetiology
- Onset commonly between 4–9 years. Bilateral in 15% cases.
- Earliest sign is a limp, usually accompanied by pain. Initial symptoms may be intermittent, causing diagnostic confusion, especially if the initial X-rays are normal.
- X-rays should be AP and frog-leg lateral. Initially the ossified portion of the femoral head appears smaller compared to its normal counterpart, together with a widened articular cartilage space. Following this the ossific nucleus becomes more radio-opaque, then the epiphysis develops a fragmented appearance. This is followed by a gradual return to normal with new bone formation.
- Differential diagnosis is inflammatory – septic arthritis, osteomyelitis, transient synovitis post-traumatic, fracture, neoplasia, slipped upper femoral capital epiphysis
- The short term aim of treatment is to reduce pain and hip stiffness
- The disease is a self limiting process and may last from 2–4 years
- Restriction of activity helps to relieve the pain, occasionally pain may be so severe as to warrant non-weight bearing with crutches and bed-rest
- The long term goal is to reduce residual deformity. Controversy exists as to the best way of doing this. The important principle is femoral head containment so that reossification produces a spherical femoral head. This can be achieved by non-operative bracing in abduction, or by operative means.
- Treatment method depends on the age of the child, severity of involvement of the femoral head and the expertise of the local orthopaedic surgeon.
- Prognosis is best for the young children, with full recovery and no disability – the remainder are left with a degree of residual disability of varying severity.

YOUR NOTES

YOUR NOTES

CHAPTER 10 – CRANIAL NERVES AND EYES

There are two main topics covered in this chapter – the cranial nerves and the eyes. They have been included together because of the considerable overlap between the two subjects. Cranial nerve examination needs to be confident and it is essential to develop an examination scheme and practise it with colleagues. It is essential also to practise and be familiar with the examination of the eyes. It is particularly important to remember that early on in eye examination some assessment of visual acuity needs to be made. Do not be caught out by a blind child. The best way to practise eye examination and to learn about the common eye conditions is to sit in on clinics with the orthoptists and ophthalmologists. In particular this will ensure you are clear about the formal assessment of visual acuity and can quickly and competently assess a squint.

SUMMARY
❑ Scheme for examination of the cranial nerves
❑ Notes on cranial nerve lesions
❑ Bulbar and pseudo-bulbar palsy
❑ Scheme for examination of the eyes
❑ Notes on the eye examination
❑ Ptosis
❑ Squint
❑ Nystagmus
❑ Fundoscopy
❑ Systemic conditions with eye signs
❑ Miscellaneous notes

SCHEME FOR EXAMINATION OF THE CRANIAL NERVES

This is a very commonly examined topic in short cases and your technique must become second nature. It is essential to practise cranial nerve examination on patients and, if necessary, on colleagues. You are unlikely to be asked to examine all the cranial nerves in one case so be prepared to test, for example, just the sixth and seventh cranial nerves.

Suggested scheme

- Enquire about sense of smell, be prepared to examine formally if requested
- Test visual acuity. Establish if the child can see (both eyes). If the child wears glasses offer to test the visual acuity with them on. This can be done grossly at the bedside by asking child to read from an age appropriate book, or to read a poster on the wall.
- Comment on any obvious abnormality such as squint and go on to examine formally if present
- Examine visual fields – sit with your face opposite the child's, one metre apart. Cover your left eye and ask child or mother to cover child's right eye. Ask child to say 'yes' when they can see your finger 'wiggling'. Move finger in from periphery at 2,5,8,11 o'clock and 'wiggle' finger. Test both eyes.
- Examine eye movements, this is really very simple as long as you remember the patient's perspective. Ask the child to follow your finger/toy with their eyes, keep the object being followed, approximately 1/2 metre from the face and the plane of movement parallel to the child's face. Keep your other hand on the child's forehead to steady it. Ask the child to tell you if they can see two. Test lateral gaze and then vertical gaze. A common pitfall is to test to the extremes of vision, where most of us will have diplopia.
- Check for nystagmus – present at extremes of gaze
- Test the sensory divisions of the trigeminal nerve (V). Ask the child to shut their eyes and to say 'yes' when they feel your touch. Gently touch the face at irregular intervals with a wisp of cotton wool, on each side, in each division of the nerve – ophthalmic, maxillary and mandibular.
- Test the motor component by asking child to close jaw tightly and palpate temporalis and masseters
- Mention corneal reflexes at the end

- Test the motor division of the facial nerve (VII). Ask the patient to raise eyebrows, puff out cheeks and smile. Look for asymmetry. Remember the sensory division which supplies the anterior 2/3 of the tongue with taste – not usually necessary to test.
- Test the auricular nerve (VIII) grossly by asking the child if they can hear a very quiet noise that you make in each ear, e.g. whisper a number the child can repeat and occlude the other ear. Offer.and know how to test formally. Ask parent about hearing.
- The glossopharyngeal nerve can be tested by the gag reflex. This should not be attempted in the exam but do mention it. Remember that the gag reflex tests the glossopharyngeal (sensory) and vagal (motor) nerves. The glossopharyngeal nerve also supplies the posterior 1/3 of the tongue with sensation.
- Test the vagal nerve by asking the child to say a short sentence. The voice will be hoarse if there is a vocal cord paralysis. The vagus can also be assessed at this point by asking the child to say 'ah' and looking at the soft palate.
- The hypoglossal nerve (XII) is tested by asking the patient to stick out their tongue and move it from side to side. Look for wasting and weakness.
- Test accessory nerve (IX) by forced rotation of the head against resistance to check for sternomastoid weakness.

At the end of the examination you should ask to

- Examine patient's glasses
- Look at fundi
- Assess pupillary responses to light and accommodation, offer to check corneal (V) and gag (IX, X) reflexes

NOTES ON CRANIAL NERVE LESIONS

Origins

III–IV mid brain
V–VIII pons
IX–XII medulla or bulb

Olfactory nerve

Traverses cribiform plate to frontal lobes, so lesions are most commonly detected in URTIs, basal skull fractures, purulent meningitis, hydrocephalus.

Optic nerve

Nerve fibres pass through optic disc to the optic nerve. Nasal fibres decussate at the chiasm and optic tracts carry impulses to the lateral geniculate bodies. The optic radiation carries the impulses to the visual cortex.

Patterns of visual defect occur, thus:

- Blindness in one eye – retinal, lens, optic nerve (chronic uveitis, optic nerve glioma, optic atrophy, septo optic dysplasia)
- Bitemporal hemianopia – craniopharyngiomas, pituitary tumours
- Homonymous hemianopia – lesions posterior to chiasm, e.g. cortical lesions such as cerebral palsy

Oculomotor nerve

Palsy is apparent as dilated pupil which faces 'down and out'. Usually congenital associated with chromosomal abnormalities or cerebral palsy. Acquired palsy may indicate tumours, infection or head injury.

Trochlear nerve

This nerve controls the superior oblique muscle. Usually presents subtly as head tilt towards the unaffected eye. On examination there is upward deviation of the eye and diplopia on downward vertical gaze. Causes include raised intracranial pressure as it has a long intracranial course. Will need surgical correction if head tilt significant.

Abducens nerve

The abducens nerve controls the lateral rectus muscle. Lesions of this nerve cause a marked convergent paralytic squint. The affected eye is turned nasally and is unable to abduct fully. Causes include raised intracranial pressure, tumours, A-V malformations, meningitis.

Trigeminal nerve

Has three sensory divisions (ophthalmic, maxillary, mandibular) which pass into the trigeminal ganglion at the apex of the petrous temporal bone. The motor fibres originate in the pons and supply the muscle of mastication.

Lesions are caused by

- Brain stem gliomas
- Infarction/arterio-venous malformation
- Acoustic neuromas
- Chronic supparative otitis media
- Cavernous sinus thrombosis

Facial nerve

The facial nerve has a long intracranial course, initially it is closely related to the sixth nerve (lesions in the pons therefore tend to affect both nerves) and it then emerges from the cerebello-pontine angle (lesions here also affect V, VI and VIII) and runs in the petrous bone in close relation to the middle ear.

An upper motor neurone lesion causes weakness of the lower part of the face on the side opposite the lesion, the forehead is spared as it is bilaterally innervated. Lower motor neurone lesions cause weakness of the whole side of the face on the same side as the lesion.

Facial palsy is a common short case in the exam.

Auditory nerve

Passes through cerebello-pontine angle (*see audiology section of development chapter*).

Glossopharyngeal, vagus and hypoglossal nerves

All leave through the jugular foramen and are affected by lesions at the base of the skull such as achondroplasia and Arnold-Chiari malformation

FACIAL NERVE PALSY

This is a very common short case.

Examination

- Smile
- Frown
- Raise the eyebrows
- Puff out the cheeks
- Whistle
- Close the eyes and keep them closed against a resistance

Lower motor neurone lesion affects the upper and lower face
Upper motor neurone lesion spares upper face

Aetiology of facial nerve palsy

LMN lesions

- Bell's palsy (by far the commonest)
- Herpes zoster (Ramsay-Hunt)
- Chronic serous otitis media
- Intracranial tumours
- Mumps
- Guillain-Barré (usually bilateral)
- Congenital – associated with obstetric forceps
- Skull fractures

UMN lesions

- Cerebral palsy
- Tumours
- Moebius' syndrome – absence of nuclei associated with bilateral sixth nerve palsies

Bell's palsy: Management

- Exclude hypertension
- Exclude other causes
- Steroids and eye drops (artificial tears)

The prognosis is generally good, better in children than in adults. All patients show signs of recovery by 4 weeks if they are going to recover.

Muscle disorders causing facial weakness

- Myotonic dystrophy
- Fascioscapulohumeral muscular dystrophy
- Congenital myopathies
- Mitochondrial myopathies
- Myasthenic syndromes

BULBAR AND PSEUDO-BULBAR PALSY

A bulbar palsy describes weakness of lower motor neurone type of the muscles supplied by the cranial nerves whose nuclei lie in the medulla (or bulb) i.e. IX–XII. It is very unusual in children.

A pseudo-bulbar palsy results from bilateral supranuclear upper motor neurone lesions of the lower cranial nerves, resulting in poor tongue and pharynx movement. This is far more common – particularly in association with spastic quadriplegia.

Signs of a pseudo-bulbar palsy

- Stiff spastic tongue which is not wasted
- 'Dry' voice and dysarthria
- Preserved gag and palatal reflexes
- Exaggerated jaw jerk

SCHEME FOR EXAMINATION OF THE EYES

- Look at the child for any obvious clues e.g. squint, ptosis, dysmorphology
- Does the child wear glasses?
- Look at the eyes – conjunctiva, pupils, lids
- Can the child see? – test both eyes – visual acuity
- Visual fields
- Eye movements
- Check for nystagmus
- Accommodation
- Pupil responses – direct and consensual light reflexes
- Cover test
- Fundoscopy

NOTES ON EYE EXAMINATION

Observation

This is very important, much pathology being visible on observation. Look first at the child. Do they look normal, are there any obvious dysmorphic features? Is the child thriving? Is the child displaying behaviour suggestive of visual impairment such as light gazing (cortical disease) or eccentric fixation with nystagmus? Look closely at the eye for squint, coloboma, corneal clouding, lesions of the iris, ptosis, anophthalmia (glass eye), microphthalmia.

The effect of glasses

This is clearly of importance and it is sensible to look at a few children with glasses on before the exam and assess their vision and the effect of glasses.

Convex glasses correct long sightedness.
Long sighted = difficulty with near vision

Concave glasses correct short sightedness.
Short sighted = difficulty with distant vision

Visual acuity

For a small child the information you will gain will be limited and should be augmented by comments about their behaviour. Check that they can fix and follow in the horizontal and vertical plane. Use an interesting but silent toy or your face. Take care to keep quiet as if you give auditory clues you will render the examination invalid.

For older children use a suitable picture or story book (age dependent – don't ask a 4-year-old to read!) for near vision and use a Snellen chart for far vision. Test both eyes separately with and without glasses (if worn).

CHECK VISION IN BOTH EYES SEPARATELY AND DON'T GET CAUGHT OUT BY UNILATERAL VISUAL LOSS

Visual fields/Eye movements/Nystagmus

See earlier

Accommodation

Ask the child to fix on your finger held in front of your face. Move your finger towards the child until it is touching the nose. Note the eye movements and pupillary responses.

Squint testing

See page 211

Pupil responses

Test direct and consensual light reflexes.

Fundoscopy

Many candidates are asked to do this and you must appear proficient. Remember to examine for the red reflex first, then examine the anterior chamber and then the fundus.

PTOSIS

This is a very common short case and you will either be invited to comment on or examine the patient's eyes.

INSTRUCTION

Examine this 12-year-old boy with ptosis.

> *This young man has a left ptosis. He is a well looking boy and there are no dysmorphic features. I would like to examine his eyes. His eyes look normal. The pupils are symmetrical. There is no obvious squint. I would like to test his vision – candidate gets him to read – vision appears normal in both eyes (tested separately). His visual fields and eye movements are normal. His direct and consensual reflexes and his ability to accommodate are normal.*

I suspect therefore that his ptosis is congenital.

Notes

The examiner will expect you to examine the eyes carefully and in doing so come up with a likely cause of the ptosis. The ptosis will become apparent on inspection. At this stage, on noting the ptosis you need to have a clear differential diagnosis in your mind.

Ptosis may be broadly classified as syndromic or neurological in origin and so it is a condition where you can earn 'points' by suggesting other systems/organs to examine.

Differential diagnosis of ptosis

- Horner's syndrome
- Third nerve palsy
- Myasthenia gravis
- Congenital

Syndromic

- Noonan's syndrome
- Rubenstein-Taybi (microcephaly, broad thumbs and toes, mental retardation)
- Smith-Lemli-Opitz
- Marcus-Gunn (aberrant innervation causes the affected lid to raise and wink when child chews or cries)

Neurological

- Third nerve palsy
- Horner syndrome
- Myasthenia gravis
- Dystrophia myotonica
- Craniosynostosis
- Neuroblastoma

Others

- Congenital (evaluate early to prevent amblyopia)
- Ocular tumours (rhabdomyosarcoma)

Features of Horner's syndrome

- Partial ptosis
- Pupil constriction
- Enophthalmus
- Ipsilateral anhydrosis
- Heterochromia iridis – indicates congenital Horner's
- Normal direct and consensual reflex

Aetiology of Horner's syndrome

- Lesion of the sympathetic nervous system in association with the brain stem, cervical cord or sympathetic plexus in association with the carotid artery

SQUINT

Examination of a squint is commonly asked in the exam and needs to be practised carefully. It is best to get an orthoptist to help you to perfect your technique.

Examination of squint

- Check the child can see first – with both eyes!
- Corneal reflections
- Eye movements
- Cover test

NOTES ON SQUINT EXAMINATION

Go straight to this after testing visual acuity. If you pick up a squint offer to test child first without and then with glasses, if prescribed. The child needs to be co-operative for this to work.

Corneal reflections

Observe both eyes whilst shining a point source of light at both corneas (corneal reflections). The light source should be held about 30 cm from the eyes and in different planes. If the eyes are straight the reflection from both corneas will be symmetrical. If there is a squint present the reflection will be asymmetrical. Beware of epicanthic folds or hypertelorism giving a false impression of squint.

Eye movements

Eye movements should be examined in all directions using an interesting object. If the eyes deviate i.e. there is asymmetry then a squint is present. If the deviation is worse in one direction then it is paralytic. If it is equal in all directions, it is non-paralytic. If it is paralytic you should be able to say which cranial nerve is involved (III,IV,VI).

The following tests should be done at near and far vision, first with glasses and then without. This avoids missing a squint caused by excessive adduction secondary to hypermetropia. Inward deviation is denoted by eso-, outward deviation exo-.

Cover/uncover test

This examines for a manifest (-tropia) squint, ask child to fix on an interesting object at 1 m and then 6 m. Cover the eye which appears to be fixing. If the other eye takes up fixation then there is a manifest squint present.

Alternate cover test

Again, ask child to fixate on an interesting object at 1 m and then 6 m. Alternately, cover each eye back and forth. Look at each eye as it is just uncovered, if it moves to take up fixation then a latent (-phoria) squint is present.

Mostly the squint will be non-paralytic.

Treatment of non-paralytic squint

There are two main aims, firstly to achieve the best possible vision in each eye. Correct any underlying defect such as cataracts or refractive errors and prevent amblyopia with occlusion therapy. Secondly, achieve the best possible ocular alignment. Surgery is commonly required.

NOTES ON PARALYTIC SQUINT

Features of a third (oculomotor) nerve lesion

- Complete ptosis
- Diplopia
- Downward and lateral gaze (unopposed lateral rectus and superior oblique muscles)
- Pupil dilatation
- Failure of the pupil to react to light or to accommodate

Features of a fourth (trochlear) nerve lesion

- Diplopia
- Failure of inferio-lateral gaze (failure of the superior oblique muscle)

Features of a sixth (abducens) nerve lesion

- Diplopia
- Medial gaze (failure of the lateral rectus muscle)

NYSTAGMUS
INSTRUCTION
Look at this boy's eyes

> **Case** – 10-year-old boy
>
> *Jack is a well looking boy who has pale skin, blue eyes and fair hair.*
> *Examination of his eyes reveals that he usually wears sunglasses, there*
> *is nystagmus and reduced visual acuity. Red reflexes are easily visible.*

I suspect he has occulocutaneous albinism

What are the long term consequences?
- Blindness and skin cancer

What is the inheritance?
- Autosomal recessive (ocular albinism alone is X-linked recessive)

NOTES ON NYSTAGMUS
- Cerebellar nystagmus is the most important type to recognise. It is usually horizontal and worsens on looking to the side of the lesion, with the fast component directed towards the side of the lesion
- Vestibular nystagmus differs in that the slow phase is directed towards the side of the lesion
- Vertical nystagmus is usually due to a lesion of the brain stem at the pontomedullary junction (roughly at the foramen magnum) e.g. achondroplasia, or Arnold-Chiari malformations
- Ocular nystagmus with slow searching movements occurs in blindness

Congenital nystagmus appears after a few months, is usually bilateral and often improves with age.

FUNDOSCOPY

NOTES ON PAPILLOEDEMA

On examination, the stages of papilloedema are

1. The optic nerve becomes hyperaemic
2. Small capillaries on optic disc disappear as they become compressed
3. Venous pulsations are no longer seen
4. The border of the optic disc becomes indistinct
5. Flame shaped haemorrhage appears around optic disc

Causes of papilloedema

- Raised intracranial pressure
- Craniopharyngioma
- Brain stem glioma
- Astrocytoma/medulloblastoma
- Leukaemia
- Infection
- Encephalopathy
- Hydrocephalus
- Intracranial haemorrhage
- Craniosynostosis
- Benign intracranial hypertension
- Hypertension
- Pseudotumour cerebri

SYSTEMIC CONDITIONS WITH EYE SIGNS

Neurofibromatosis	Lisch nodule, ptosis
Wilson's disease	Kayser-Fleischer ring
Ataxia telangiectasia	Conjunctival telangiectasia
Down's syndrome	Brushfield spots – not pathognomonic
Hyperthyroidism	Exophthalmos, lid lag
Juvenile chronic arthritis	Iridocyclitis

Causes of a cherry red spot

- Tay-Sach's disease
- Niemann-Pick disease
- GM1 gangliosidosis
- Sanhoff disease
- Mucolipidosis

Causes of lens dislocation

- Marfan's
- Homocystinuria
- Ehlers-Danlos syndrome

Causes of cataracts

- Metabolic disease galactosaemia
- Wilson's disease
- Hypopararthyroidism
- Diabetes
- Dystrophica myotonica

Causes of corneal clouding

- GM1 gangliosidosis
- Fucosidosis
- Mucopolysaccharidosis
- Mucolipidosis

Causes of coloboma

- Aniridia – Wilm's association
- CHARGE association
- Goldenhar syndrome
- Inherited – autosomal dominant

MISCELLANEOUS NOTES

Marfan's syndrome

Lens dislocation is present in 80% of adults and 50% of 5 year olds with Marfan's syndrome. It usually dislocates superiorly and temporally. Symptoms include blurred vision, due to refractive changes and diplopia. If the pupil is dilated the edge of the lens may be seen as a black crescent on ophthalmoscopic examination. A clearer view is obtained with slit lamp examination.

Duane's syndrome

A congenital abnormality of innervation causing simultaneous contraction of medial and lateral recti on attempted adduction of the affected eye. On examination they may have exo- or eso-tropia, and on testing eye movements they may have failure to abduct or adduct the affected eye.

Moebius' syndrome

This is manifest as a (usually) bilateral but asymmetrical LMN facial nerve palsy, associated with sixth nerve palsies which cause failure of abduction and paralytic convergent squints of the affected eyes. The cause is unknown, but as both cranial nerves are closely related it may be due to underdevelopment of the cranial nerve nuclei.

Ramsay Hunt syndrome

This is an eruption of herpes zoster vesicles on the posterior wall of the ear canal accompanied by a LMN facial nerve palsy. Spontaneous recovery is the rule.

Uveitis

This is inflammation of the uveal tract consisting of the inner vascular coat of the eye, the iris, the ciliary body and choroid. Iritis may occur alone or in conjunction with the ciliary body as irido-cyclitis. This commonly occurs insidiously without symptoms and for this reason children with seropositive (ANA) arthritis have to have regular eye review.

Case – 8-year-old girl

Jane is a well looking girl. She appears Cushingoid. Examination of her eyes reveals conjunctival injection. The visual acuity of her left eye is markedly reduced. It was not possible to examine the visual fields. The pupil responses are present but slow on the left. Ophthalmoscopy reveals clouding of the cornea on the left.

This would fit with chronic uveitis. I would like to proceed to a full systemic examination, paying particular attention to the joints and looking for the side-effects of steroids.

YOUR NOTES

YOUR NOTES

YOUR NOTES

CHAPTER 11 – CHILD DEVELOPMENT

It is essential to revise development and acquire the skills to assess children's development confidently in the exam looking as if you have done it before! This needs practice. You need to attend child development clinics, visual assessment clinics and audiological clinics and need to liaise with your local community paediatricians to ensure you get this experience. Some basic background information and a list of potential scenarios you may meet are included in this chapter. Refer also to the further reading in the back of the book. It is important to learn some milestones and to know the details of and be confident in performing more specialist assessment of vision and hearing.

Development is a continuous process from conception to maturity and depends on myelination of the nervous system. The sequence of events is the same for all children, it is the rate of development that varies. Primitive reflexes must be lost before voluntary movement can develop. Remember that development is a cephalocaudal process, beginning with the acquisition of head control moving down through the neck and back with sitting and the development of hand movements to the legs and the acquisition of leg control and walking. Also, generalised mass movement gives way to individual responses.

When assessing development in the examination, remember that it is generally split up into gross motor, fine motor and vision, speech and hearing and social. Although they are obviously not mutually exclusive, it is best to present your findings in terms of the four groups. By thinking of them individually, you should be able to determine if development is normal or delayed, and if it is delayed, is it globally delayed or delayed in one particular area e.g. motor delay in a child with a hemiplegia. You only have a short time and a full sophisticated developmental assessment is not possible. No-one will expect you to perform a full Griffith's assessment in 5 minutes!

SUMMARY

- Stages of development and milestones
- Scenarios   6 months
  - 12 months
  - 2½ years
  - Pre-school
- Bottom shuffling

- Down's syndrome
- Visual assessment
- Assessment of hearing
- Education Act
- Children Act

Helpful hints – Observe the child carefully before jumping in.

1. Take a good look at the child, are they obviously dysmorphic, or have they, for example got a hemiplegia or other neurological problem?
2. Go with the child. If they are playing when you are introduced to them, watch what they are doing for a short while and comment on that first e.g. playing with a pencil and paper, how are they holding the pencil, what are they drawing, what shapes are they making. In the first few seconds you will already have an idea of fine motor skills of the child.
3. Get down to the child's level and play with them, don't make them play for you. If they are performing a task and you wish to move on to something else, gently introduce the new task. Do not take away all the other things the child was playing with and then force them do what you want them to – they won't, you'll have lost their attention and they will not play the game any more!
4. When assessing them at any level, see what they do spontaneously first and then see if you can get the child to perform at the next stage up e.g. scribbling vertical lines, can they imitate a circle, walking, can they run etc. This gives you a better idea of their exact stage of development. It is very important not to ask the child to do things they are unlikely to achieve e.g. ask a 2 year old to draw a circle.
5. Be prepared to ask the parent questions (ask the permission of the examiners) particularly about vision, hearing and social development.
6. Most importantly try to gain the confidence of the child and be nice to them. It will be appreciated by the child, the parent and the examiners.

STAGES OF DEVELOPMENT
Remember the areas of development

- Gross motor
- Fine motor and vision
- Speech and hearing
- Social

When assessing children information from each of these areas is required.

Developmental milestones

This is not meant to be a detailed list, these can be found in many different textbooks, this is a simple outline. We would suggest you learn a list of milestones similar to that below.

6 WEEKS

Gross motor	holds chin up when prone, beginning to lose head lag
Fine motor and vision	follows object up to 180 degrees in the horizontal plane, watches people
Social	smiles

12 WEEKS

Gross motor	lifts head and chest with extended arms when prone, reaches forward, but misses objects, supine early head control, loss of Moro reflex, makes defensive movements
Fine motor and vision	fixes and follows in the horizontal and vertical plane
Social	sustained social contact, listens to music, begins to vocalise

16 WEEKS

Gross motor	lifts head and chest into vertical axis, legs extended, hands in midline, reaches and grasps objects and brings them to the mouth. No head lag on pulling to the sitting position. Held erect, pushes with feet.
Social	laughs out loud, shows displeasure, excited at sight of food

28 WEEKS

Gross motor	rolls over prone to supine (first) then supine to prone, sits with rounded back and leans forward on hands, supports most of weight on standing and bounces actively, reaches out and grasps for large objects, transfers from hand to hand, grasps using radial grasp, rakes at pellets
Speech and hearing	polysyllabic vowel sounds formed
Social	prefers mother, babbles, enjoys mirror

40 WEEKS

Gross motor	sits alone without support, back straight, pulls to standing position and cruises around the furniture, creeps and crawls
Fine motor and vision	grasps objects with thumb and forefinger, pokes at things with a forefinger, picks up a pellet with assisted pincer grip (using radial border of arm), uncovers hidden toy, object permanence
Speech and hearing	repetitive consonant sounds mama, dada, should pass distraction test (see later)
Social	responds to sound of name, plays peek-a-boo or pat-a-cake, waves bye-bye

1 YEAR

Gross motor	walks with one hand held, rises independently
Fine motor and vision	full pincer grip, releases objects on request
Speech and hearing	few words besides mama, dada, beginning to have meaning
Social	plays simple ball game, makes postural adjustments to dressing

15 MONTHS

Gross motor	walks alone, crawls upstairs
Fine motor and vision	makes tower 3 cubes, makes line with crayon, inserts pellet into bottle
Speech and hearing	jargon, may name familiar objects
Social	hugs parents, indicates desires and needs

18 MONTHS

Gross motor	runs stiffly, sits on small chair, walks upstairs with hand held, explores
Fine motor and vision	tower of 4 cubes, imitates scribbling, imitates vertical strokes, dumps pellet
Speech and hearing	10 words, names pictures, identifies one or more body parts
Social	feeds self, seeks help, tells when wet/soiled, kisses parents with pucker

2 YEARS

Gross motor	runs well, walks up and down stairs one step at a time, opens doors, climbs on furniture, jumps
Fine motor and vision	tower 7 cubes, circular scribbling, imitates horizontal strokes
Speech and hearing	puts 3 words together (subject, verb, object)
Social	handles spoon well, listens to stories, tells immediate experiences, helps to undress

2½ YEARS

Gross motor	upstairs alternating feet
Fine motor and vision	tower 9 cubes, vertical and horizontal strokes but not yet a cross, forms closed figure
Speech and hearing	refers to self as I, uses proper name
Social	helps put things away, pretends in play

3 YEARS

Gross motor	rides tricycle, stands on one foot momentarily
Fine motor and vision	tower 10 cubes, imitates bridge of 3 cubes, copies circle, imitates cross
Speech and hearing	knows age and sex, counts 3 objects correctly, repeats 3 numbers
Social	plays simple games in parallel with other children, helps in dressing, washes hands

4 YEARS

Gross motor	hops on one foot, throws ball over hand, uses scissors to cut out picture, climbs well
Fine motor and vision	copies bridge from model, imitates construction of gate from 5 cubes, copies cross and square, draws a man with 2 to 4 parts without the head
Speech and hearing	counts 4 pennies accurately, tells a story
Social	plays with other children with beginning of social interaction, goes to toilet alone

5 YEARS

Gross motor	skips
Fine motor and vision	draws triangle from copy, names heavier of 2 weights
Speech and hearing	names 4 colours, repeats sentence of 10 syllables, counts 10 pennies correctly
Social	dresses and undresses, asks questions about the meaning of words, domestic role-playing

SCENARIOS

- **Six-month-old – Assess this child's development**
- **Twelve-month-old – Assess this child's development**
- **2½ years – Assess this child's development**
- **Pre-school children – Assess this child's development**

Whenever approaching any of these situations you will get the most information by observing the child. This will give you a starting point for at least their gross motor skills and often their fine motor skills as well. Be careful when changing the child from one task to another and give them enough time to show you what they can do. When appropriate, ask mother to manoeuvre the child, it will cause them less distress. Chat with the child and its mother. It is reasonable, particularly with the older child, to ask the parent one or two questions.

These scenarios are notes to get you started and focus mainly on the gross motor, fine motor and vision. Assessment of speech and hearing and social development is also needed in some detail. The milestones must be known. Information on the assessment of hearing is covered later. Make appropriate comments, for example if the child is alert, interested and playful, say so.

SIX MONTH OLD – ASSESS THIS CHILD'S DEVELOPMENT

Gross motor – observe at bedside

- Sitting on parent's lap, comment on sitting position, straightness of back (at this stage should be sitting with support but straight back), will they sit unsupported (next stage up)?
- Ask mother to lie them prone, observe, at 6 months should be able to lift head and chest clear, supporting weight on extended arms
- Do they roll, if so, both ways? If do not demonstrate ask the examiner if you can ask the mother if they can
- Lie them supine, are they able to lift head up, do they grab their feet
- Hold standing, do they take their weight

Fine motor and vision

- Offer an object, should pick it up with a palmar grasp (next stage is holding in a mature grip between thumb and index finger)
- How long do they hold the object, at 6 months will hold for short period and then drop with no object permanence and carry on unaware they have dropped it
- Do they transfer hand to hand, should at 6 months
- Offer second object, at 6 months will either ignore the second object, or drop the first object and take the second object (next stage is developing object permanence and hence try to hold first object and take second)

Speech and hearing

- Are they vocalising, are there any concerns about hearing?

Social

- Do they put the object in their mouth. Are they smiling, laughing and alert? Do they fix on their mother's face?

TWELVE MONTH OLD – ASSESS THIS CHILD'S DEVELOPMENT

Gross motor

- Observe at the bedside and comment
- Are they sitting unsupported?
- Ask mother to lie them prone, do they raise themselves to the sitting position, and from the sitting position do they start to crawl on all fours?
- When placed against furniture, do they pull themselves to standing position and begin to cruise around the furniture?
- Can they stand alone?

Fine motor and vision

- Offer them some small objects, e.g. paper pieces, hundreds and thousands etc. Do they pick them up with a mature pincer grip?
- Ask mother if they feed themselves or hold their bottle
- Do they cast toys deliberately and watch them fall to the ground?
- If given 2 objects do they bring them to the midline and perhaps bang them together?

Speech and hearing
- Do they know any words with meaning, are there any concerns about hearing? Be prepared to do a distraction test, if asked.

Social
- Do they imitate clapping their hands and waving bye-bye?
- Are they speaking, ask mother if they are saying appropriate words
- Ask mother if they will help with dressing

2½ YEARS – ASSESS THIS CHILD'S DEVELOPMENT

Gross motor
- Observe their play
- Are they walking, can they easily squat and come up from that position?
- Can they run?
- Ask mother if they walk upstairs without holding on, how do they come downstairs
- Can they jump with both feet together?
- Can they imitate standing on tiptoe?

Fine motor and vision
- How many bricks do they build in a block, should be 7
- Can they build a train with 3 bricks?
- Give them a pen and paper, do they imitate a circle and a horizontal line (next stage can draw circle and line without demonstration)?
- Can they manipulate pegs into a peg board, simple jigsaws if available?

Speech and hearing
- Can they speak in short sentences, is the speech clear, are there any concerns about hearing?

Social
- Can they feed themselves, help with dressing/undressing, tell parents when wet/dry, kiss and socialise?

PRE-SCHOOL CHILD – ASSESS THIS CHILD'S DEVELOPMENT

Gross motor and vision

- Approx. 5 years
- Can they skip, and jump lightly on their toes?
- Can they walk heel to toe?
- Ask mother if they climb, slide and swing
- Can they catch a ball?

Fine motor and vision

- Copy a square and a triangle, house with a door, windows, roof, and a chimney
- Can they construct a gate?
- Can they recognise and copy letters from the alphabet?

Speech and hearing

- Speech should be confident, can they name colours, can they count to 10, are there any concerns about hearing?

Social

- Play games with more complicated rules
- Can they tell the time, recognise letters and numbers and begin to read?

MISCELLANEOUS NOTES

Bottom shuffling

This runs in families and tends to delay walking, bottom shufflers often not walking until 18–24 months. There is no evidence that bottom shuffling itself delays development in any other way, hence it is important to establish, in a child who is over 18 months old, not walking but bottom shuffling, their locomotor skills. Bottom shuffle is usually an isolated event and and such children will eventually walk, although a careful look is required as hemiplegic children often bottom shuffle.

If they bottom shuffle, it is usually an isolated event and they will eventually walk although a careful look is required as for example, hemiplegic children often bottom shuffle.

Down's syndrome

The common misconception is that Down's syndrome children are grossly developmentally delayed. There is a complete spectrum of disabilities of Down's syndrome and the disability tends to be a learning disability rather than a physical disability. In the first few years development can often be normal, with learning problems becoming apparent at 3–4 years. In view of this their educational placement should depend on their ability rather than their diagnosis – some Down's syndrome children enjoy integration into mainstream education, although most will eventually require some form of more specialised provision. When faced with a Down's syndrome child for a developmental assessment, do not be put off, the developmental examination is just the same, and they may fall within the normal range for motor development.

VISUAL ASSESSMENT

The chapter on cranial nerves and eyes should be read. It is essential to watch experts assess vision. These are some additional notes on the assessment of visual acuity.

Assessing visual acuity

Most of the time this is fulfilled by observation. Observe the ability to fix and follow and then later to pick up small objects at the peripheries of the visual field in the younger child. In the older child use a picture book or the written word. Remember to test both eyes. It is of crucial importance to stay quiet when assessing vision so as not to use voice as the stimulus. The examiner will look for this. I have seen numerous candidates slip up on this.

It is also essential to have some background which relates to the more sophisticated assessment of visual acuity.

- Minimum observable tests where you attempt to establish the smallest object the child can see e.g. hundreds and thousands, silver sweets, smarties, cubes or the Stycar graded balls.

- Minimum separable tests measuring the ability to separate visual stimuli and forming the most precise method e.g. Snellen charts (not under 3 years), Stycar letter tests, Stycar toy tests, Sonksen-Silver test, silhouettes, Ladybird pictures, forced choice preferential looking acuity card procedure.

- Whichever method is used, each eye should be tested separately. This is well tolerated <8 months and >2 years but not inbetween. The eye should be covered with the parent's hand, a patch or a blackened lens. Most children will co-operate with both eyes open up to the age of 3 years, but will not co-operate with covering the eye until about 4 years.

Electrophysiological techniques are useful in the investigation of some visual disorders, particularly the inherited retinal disorders, cerebral storage diseases and demyelinating diseases.

- Electroretinogram (ERG) is derived from the outer or superficial layers of the retina and may be normal when there is complete optic atrophy, or completely abnormal when there is retinitis pigmentosa long before a clinical defect becomes apparent.

- Visual evoked responses represent the electrophysiological activity generated when the nerve impulses travel from the eye to the cortex, and is used to assess the integrity of the visual pathways. It is useful when used in conjunction with the ERG.

ASSESSMENT OF HEARING

It is essential to attend an audiology clinic to learn about the assessment of hearing. The information in this section is intended as helpful notes and should be read in conjunction with standard texts and practical experience gained in the clinic setting.

- 0.5–1 newborn/1000 live births have permanent, moderate to severe, bilateral sensorineural hearing loss. In addition children become deaf throughout childhood for various reasons, and the estimated prevalence of permanent, bilateral hearing loss of moderate to severe degree increases to 1.5–2/1000 children under the age of 6 years.
- Important as a screening procedure; hearing tests are performed in all children at some stage, as deafness can have a major impact on the development of the child. The earlier the defect is picked up the better the prognosis.
- Until children reach the developmental age of 3–4 years, they cannot be expected to respond to a pure tone audiogram, so different methods of assessment must be employed.
- You should not be asked to perform a hearing test in the exam as you will soon learn that examination rooms (which contain a lot of children) have a background noise level far above that acceptable for a hearing test. You may be asked to talk the examiner through one of the general principles.
- There are 2 types of hearing tests, those used for the diagnosis of hearing loss, and those used as screening procedures.
- Good history from the parents is the first step in a hearing assessment – parental suspicion of hearing loss, family history, high risk factors, failed screening test, symptoms of middle ear disease or behavioural problems.

Distraction testing

- By 6–9 months, children have learnt to control their sitting balance and head posture and can turn to sound either above or behind them, hence they can take part in a distraction test.
- Explain the test to the mother/carer
- Position the baby carefully
- The distractor sits in front of the baby and gains their attention by any appropriate means

- This activity is then suddenly stopped, the baby waits for the reintroduction of play and the tester, who is standing behind the baby and out of their visual field, presents a sound stimulus
- When the baby turns to look for the sound source they are rewarded with praise. If they do not respond, the tester raises the intensity of the sound stimulus until the baby responds.
- Sounds are presented to each side
- Pitfalls: the baby becomes too interested in the examiner or baby responds to visual stimulus after play has ceased and becomes used to the test.

Distraction with visual reinforcement
- Some audiology rooms are equipped with loud speakers through which a variety of electronically controlled signals can be played in a sophisticated version of the distraction test.

Co-operative tests
- Distraction testing becomes more difficult after 15 months as the child develops object permanence and becomes more engrossed in play (they are unlikely to turn to even loud noises in the distraction test)
- From this stage onwards it is usually possible to use co-operative tests, although the age range at which children will co-operate is wide
- Here you use either the child's ability to discriminate speech or tasks that demand a response to certain sounds
- One of each should usually be performed
- It is difficult to assess each ear separately, but to a certain extent this is academic as the immediate aim is to assess functional hearing and the ability to develop language.

Speech discrimination tests

- The McCormick toy test is the most widely used. Here a set of toys are placed in front of the child. Generally they are paired, with each pair having similar sounding names e.g. key and tree, cup and duck, horse and house, spoon and shoe etc. Having involved the child in play with these toys, the examiner covers their mouth (to stop the child lip reading), and lowers the level of their voice intensity and asks the child to identify one of the objects on the table.
- The voice should be at a level of 30–40 dB

Performance tests

- In these tests the child is asked to perform a particular task when they hear a certain sound (e.g. placing a brick in a basket)
- The child must not be able to see the examiner making the test noise
- The sound stimulus may be warble tones or narrow band noise at varying levels of intensity
- The child must be familiar with the game first

Pure tone audiometry

- Pure tone audiogram is a reliable method of testing children in each ear and can be consistently used in the normal child from 5 years onwards, sometimes earlier
- Headphones are placed on the child and they are started with an easily audible tone, gradually reducing until the tone can no longer be heard
- Each ear is tested in turn
- Pitfalls: uncooperative children, unintentional visual clues by the tester or the parent
- Anxious children may not respond to the sound even at high levels
- This should be cross-checked with formal or informal speech tests

Electrical response audiometry

- These tests are based on the fact that a few milliseconds after sound reaches the ear, action potentials are propagated in the cochlea, along the auditory pathways to the brainstem and cortex
- It is possible to detect these potentials and use them to find the child's threshold for hearing

Brain stem auditory evoked responses

- The BSER is recorded from 3 surface electrodes (usually scalp, mastoid and forehead). It represents the transmission of the auditory signal from the cochlea to the brainstem.
- The child can be awake (if very relaxed), asleep or under anaesthetic
- The complex waveform is demonstrated by computer analysis of the EEG
- It is particularly useful for children who are autistic, blind or severely learning disabled and widely used as a screening test in high risk neonates

Evoked otoacoustic emissions

- Sound stimulus produces an acoustic emission from the cochlea which can be detected by a small microphone placed within the ear canal, analysed and displayed, the child needs to be calm and still
- Any hearing defect, even a minor conductive defect abolishes this, and hence this is a very good test both for screening and diagnosis
- It does not however establish the degree of hearing loss

Electrocochleography

- A needle electrode is inserted through the tympanic membrane, on to the promontory of the middle ear, and the action potentials of the cochlea are recorded
- The stimulus is normally a train of clicks
- A general anaesthetic is usually required and this invasive test is rarely used

SCREENING FOR HEARING LOSS

- The need for early detection of hearing defects is clear and screening for hearing loss is carried out in all infants in the UK
- The traditional way of performing this is by the distraction test at 6–9 months, usually carried out by health visitors
- The test is satisfactory and reliable but the level of continued training and supervision is high
- Its value as a screening test for the hearing loss associated with secretory otitis media is also limited as this condition evolves throughout childhood
- It remains the most widely used screening test at present
- Selective screening of high risk neonates for sensori-neural deafness is by BSER or OAE (see page 237). Suitable groups include preterm infants, FH of hearing loss, consanguinuity, dysmorphic syndromes, suspected or proven maternal intrauterine infections
- By testing all such infants 40–60% of all congenital hearing loss can be detected. There is considerable interest in the establishment of universal screening for sensori-neural deafness in the neonatal period by otoacoustic emissions.
- A high degree of vigilance by professionals dealing with children and parents is an additional and excellent screening test
- Children at school entry undergo a hearing test in the form of a simplified PTA (pure tone audiogram) at a fixed intensity, usually 20–25 dB. Any failing the assessment are referred to an audiological clinic.

NOTES ON THE EDUCATION ACT

- Introduced in 1981 and updated in 1993
- Thrust was towards integration of 'physically and mentally handicapped' children into mainstream schools
- It was assumed that most children's special needs could be met in mainstream schools, with some children requiring additional facilities and resources
- The children who are thought likely to have the most need for additional provision are to be the subject of an assessment
- At the end of the assessment, the local education authority decide whether or not to issue a document which is legally binding, known as the statement of special educational needs
- Either the health authority, the education authority or the parents can ask for an assessment under the Education Act
- This assessment includes asking for reports from the child's nursery or school, from social services departments, a medical report, a report from any other professionals known to be involved with the child and from the parents
- It is initiated and co-ordinated by the local education authority
- All these reports are then collated by the LEA and turned into a final provisional statement which must be shown to the parents before it is passed. The parents have the right to appeal if they are not satisfied.
- The LEA then makes the decision as to whether a statement is produced (some children have all the reports etc. submitted and are not considered eligible for a statement)
- The LEA makes the decision as to how and where to provide for each child's special needs, whether that be mainstream schools or special schools
- The statemented pupils, whether in mainstream or special schools, should be reviewed annually with their parents, and there is a statutory reassessment of all statemented pupils between the ages of 13½ years and 14½ years
- The children who receive educational statements vary widely from the physically handicapped, who usually come to light in the pre-school years, to the behaviourally disturbed, to the mentally handicapped, to the children who require extra help as they fall behind their peers.

NOTES ON THE CHILDREN ACT

- Introduced in 1989 and came into force in October 1991
- Essentially, it places the welfare of the child above all other considerations and aims to strike a balance between family independence and the protection of the child
- It is based upon the belief that most children are best looked after within the family without unwarranted interference. Parental responsibilities replace the former concept of parents' rights.
- It prevents the implementation of any court order on the child unless it contributes positively to the child's welfare
- Children who are looked after by the local authority must be consulted before decisions are made about matters affecting them. In addition to promoting their welfare, regard must be given to race, religion, culture and language. Contact with families and friends must be promoted unless it is inconsistent with their welfare.
- It makes local authorities responsible for the provision of services for children in need. Under the act, a child (considered to be an individual under the age of 18) is considered to be in need if:
  - they are unlikely to achieve or maintain, or have the opportunity of achieving or maintaining, a reasonable standard of health or development without the provision of services
  - their health or development is likely to be significantly impaired, or further impaired, without the provision of such services
  - they are disabled

Health = physical or mental health; development = physical, intellectual, emotional, social or behavioural development.
- Every local authority should hold a register of children with needs, most noticeably a child protection register and a register for children with disabilities
- The children's act also outlines a series of orders for the protection of children who are 'at risk'.

Care and supervision orders

- The care order places the child in the care of the local authority and confers the parental responsibility on the authority
- The supervision order places the child under the supervision of the local authority or a probation officer and may impose conditions such as a medical or psychiatric examination
- A care order, unless it is revised, lasts until the child is 18 years; a supervision order remains in force for 1 year initially

Emergency protection orders (EPO)

- Short term order and can be applied for by anyone, although in practice the local authority or NSPCC is usually involved
- It lasts for 8 days, can be renewed for a further 7 days and can be appealed at 3 days
- It gives the applicant parental responsibility
- Replaced the place of safety order

Child assessment order

- New order, granted in non-urgent circumstances, where the suspicion is that the child is suffering, or likely to suffer, significant harm, but where the investigation to establish the facts requires assessment which is refused by the parents or carers
- Requires child to be produced for assessment and lasts for 7 days

Police protection provisions

- Any police constable can take a child into police protection for up to 3 days without assuming parental responsibility.

YOUR NOTES

YOUR NOTES

YOUR NOTES

CHAPTER 12 – NEUROLOGY

Neurology is a difficult area to provide information on how to assess cases in the exam. There is a very large amount of potential information including considerable background information on specific subjects. We have confined ourselves principally to discussion of the potential scenarios you are likely to meet in the exam. We would recommend further reading of neurological examination as the information presented is intended to be a summary.

SUMMARY

- ❑ Scheme for examination of peripheral nervous system
- ❑ Scheme for examination of gait
- ❑ Sensory examination
- ❑ Scheme for cerebellar examination
- ❑ Abnormalities of posture and movement
- ❑ Useful lists
- ❑ Cerebral palsy
- ❑ Neuromuscular disease
- ❑ Ataxia
- ❑ Spina bifida
- ❑ Neurocutaneous syndromes

SCHEME FOR EXAMINATION OF THE PERIPHERAL MOTOR SYSTEM

This needs to be done carefully and correctly. It is essential to practise and make your technique second nature. Remember to look for obvious clues first (e.g. obvious neurological deficit such as cerebral palsy, orthoses, wheelchairs). The examiner may limit you to the arms or the legs. You should have a different approach to infants and older children.

Infants

Most information is gained by observation and so spend some time watching and playing with the infant. Try to get eye contact – see if the child will fix and follow in the horizontal and vertical plane. Look for any obvious dysmorphology. A baby lifting their right arm has at least grade 3 power in that limb. Look specifically for leg scissoring (spastic diplegia), paucity of movement on one side (hemiplegia), overall paucity of movement (spinal muscular atrophy).

Perform a brief neurodevelopmental assessment. It is essential to know the normal milestones (*see development chapter*).

- Pull the child to sit – use one hand to pull up both hands and the other to support the head
- Hold the child by the trunk in the sitting position
- Assess standing posture
- Hold the child up prone looking at tone and head control
- Place the child on the bed prone to see if the child supports its head, supports itself on its forearms (3 months) or outstretched hands (6 months)
- Proceed with further examination dependent upon the initial findings

Remember that if the head is extended when the child is held prone that this may reflect extensor spasm. Head control is better assessed by pulling the child to sit.

Proceed to examine the tendon reflexes as you would in an older child. Examine for ankle clonus (one or two beats are normal under one year), plantars (up going until one year).

Ask the mother about hand preference, which is abnormal under one year.

Finally, examine for the presence of the primitive reflexes. e.g. Moro, asymmetric tonic neck reflex, grasp etc.

Older children

This should be done more conventionally as older children can co-operate. Ask the child to walk first unless there is an obvious reason why they cannot (e.g. in a wheelchair). Look for clues as above.

- Look at muscle bulk, symmetry and for scars e.g. tendo-achilles shortening
- Examine tone – include testing for clonus
- Examine power
- Examine reflexes
- Further examination as appropriate

UPPER MOTOR NEURONE OR LOWER MOTOR NEURONE LESION

This relatively straightforward piece of information is often asked for. It is very important to be ready for this question with the correct answer as a number of candidates when asked this do not appreciate what information the examiner is requesting.

Characteristics of an upper motor neurone lesion

- Increased tone
- Clonus
- Reduced power
- Increased reflexes

Characteristics of a lower motor neurone lesion

- Wasting
- Fasciculation
- Reduced tone
- Reduced power
- Reduced reflexes

SCHEME FOR EXAMINATION OF GAIT

The examination of gait is very important and often asked. The question can either be a direct one or phrased indirectly such as examine this child's legs when, providing the child can walk, gait examination is the appropriate first step.

Abnormalities to be looked for are

- Hemiplegia
- Diplegia
- Ataxia
- Neuromuscular disease
- Orthopaedic problems
- Rheumatological disorders

Children with abnormal gaits need to be viewed (try child development unit or general outpatients) so that you have seen common abnormalities and are able to spot them in the exam. It is sensible to use a scheme for examination and one is suggested below.

General points

First check with the child or parents that they can walk. Look at the child Do they look dysmorphic, is there an obvious cerebral palsy, is there a built up shoe, are there sticks or a wheelchair nearby?

Spastic gait

Ask the child to walk unaided – look at arm and leg movement for signs of a hemiplegia. The arm will be flexed on the affected side. If you suspect hemiplegia ask the child to walk fast or walk on tip toe which will make the neurology more pronounced. Continue looking – are the legs stiff and abducted, if so a diplegia is likely, a diplegia will also become more pronounced if you ask the child to walk fast or on tip toe.

- If the child has either a hemiplegia or a diplegia you can then take the child to the examination couch and confirm the neurology with a careful peripheral neurological examination.
- You may then be asked if you want to examine anywhere else – upper limbs, cranial nerves, skin (neurocutaneous syndrome).

Ataxic gait

If the gait is not spastic the next thing to consider is whether it is ataxic (unsteady and broad based). Ask the child to heel to toe walk (you will need to demonstrate this). If the child is ataxic this will be difficult. Then ask the child to stand still (should fall over towards the side of a cerebellar lesion). Ask the child to close their eyes. If the lesion is cerebellar there should be no deterioration. If the ataxia is as a consequence of a dorsal column problem the child will fall (Romberg's sign). The latter is rare in childhood.

- If you feel the gait is ataxic and due to a cerebellar lesion confirm this with a cerebellar examination (see later).

Neuromuscular problem

The next possibility is that you are dealing with either a neuromuscular or a lower motor neurone problem. Look for a waddling gait and foot drop. Examine for Gower's sign.

- If the Gower's sign is positive a peripheral neurological examination should be carried out and the back checked for a scoliosis or spina bifida.

Others

Finally, consider either an orthopaedic or a rheumatological problem.

NOTES ON EXAMINATION OF GAIT

Gower's sign

Ask the child to sit on the floor and then stand up without using the hands for assistance. A positive Gower's is when the child rises from the floor by pushing off, and crawling up his legs with his hands, to overcome proximal pelvic weakness.

Limp

The aetiology of limp is divided into two groups.

- **Painful limp** is also known as an antalgic gait. Here the child spends the least amount of time possible on the affected limb. This is Trendelenburg negative which implies the affected hip is higher than the unaffected hip.
- **Non-painful limp** is also known as a Trendelenburg gait. Here the child shifts their centre of gravity over the affected side for balance and is an indicator of proximal muscle weakness or hip instability. Trendelenburg positive implies the affected hip is lower than the unaffected hip.

There are many different causes of a limp which change with different age groups. Some examples are listed below.

Antalgic	Infection
	Trauma
	Perthes' disease
	Rheumatological (juvenile chronic arthritis)
Trendelenburg	Congenital hip dislocation
	Neurological (muscular dystrophy)
	Slipped capital femoral epiphysis

SENSORY EXAMINATION

This would be very difficult in the context of the exam. Your approach to the child will be important and you need to encourage co-operation to gain maximum information. For older children you should have a polished technique so that you not only put the child at ease, but are able to concentrate on the signs elicited.

Pain, light touch and temperature	Spinothalamic tracts
Joint position sense, vibration and proprioception	Posterior columns

ATAXIA

Ataxia is the incoordination that results from either sensory loss or cerebellar dysfunction. In children the latter cause is by far the most common.

Romberg's sign

The child is asked to stand with the feet just sufficiently apart to become steady. The child then closes the eyes. If the child has a cerebellar problem there is no deterioration in balance. If the child has a sensory ataxia then he or she will fall.

SCHEME FOR CEREBELLAR EXAMINATION

There is no definite order to do this. Fortunately it is rarely called upon. However if asked to examine the cerebellar function you need to have your own scheme. Below is a suggested scheme.

Start by observing the gait which is ataxic and broad based, leaning towards the side of the lesion if unilateral.

- Test eye movements and look for nystagmus – horizontal and maximal looking to the side of the lesion
- Ask the child a question and listen for dysarthria
- Test coordination. Ask the child to touch his finger then your nose with his index finger. Look for past pointing or intention tremor. Assess rapidly alternating movements (dysdiadochokinesis)
- Examine the arms and legs for hypotonia and hyporeflexia
- Ask the child to sit to check for truncal ataxia
- Stand the child up and examine for Romberg's sign to differentiate sensory posterior column disease from cerebellar
- Think of the causes of ataxia and look for associated signs e.g. telangiectasia or pes cavus

ABNORMALITIES OF POSTURE AND MOVEMENT

Tremor

- Physiological
- Drug induced – salbutamol, thyroxine
- Benign essential tremor – positive family history, intentional
- Cerebellar – not present at rest, intentional
- Parkinson's (rare) – present at rest (not intentional)

Myotonia

- The failure of muscle to relax after contraction

Dystonia

- Abnormal posturing of the limbs, trunk and face
- Can occur in association with choreoathetosis
- e.g. cerebral palsy, drug induced, Wilson's disease

Chorea

- Rapid irregular repetitive jerking, either generalised or affecting one part of the body

Athetosis

- Slow writhing movement of the limbs

Dystonia and choreoathetosis are abnormalities of posture and movement secondary to extrapyramidal dysfunction.

Case

John is a 12-year-old boy in a wheelchair. He is mentally alert but has posturing dystonic with choreoathetoid movements. The diagnosis is cerebral palsy and likely causes of the cerebral palsy include perinatal asphyxia or kernicterus.

Tic

- A sudden brief and purposeless stereotyped movement which can, to at least some extent, be suppressed by voluntary effort

USEFUL LISTS

Reflexes	Spinal segment	Nerve
Biceps	C5,6	musculocutaneous
Supinator or brachioradialis jerk	C5,6	radial
Triceps	C6,7	radial
Superficial abdominal	T7-12	
Knee	L234	femoral
Ankle	S1	tibial
Plantars	S1	

Spinal levels of some cutaneous reflexes

Superficial abdominal	T7-12
Cremasteric	L1
Plantar	S1
Anal	S4-5

MRC grading of power

0   No contraction
1   Flicker or trace of contraction
2   Active movement with gravity eliminated
3   Active movement against gravity
4   Active movement against gravity and resistance
5   Normal power

Myotomes

Movement tested	Nerve root
Shoulder abduction	C5/6
Elbow flexion	C5/6
Elbow extension	C7/8
Finger flexion	C8
Finger abduction	C8/T1
Hip flexion	L1
Hip adduction	L2
Knee extension	L3
Foot dorsiflexion	L4
Foot plantar flexion	S1
Knee flexion	S2
Hip flexion	S3

CEREBRAL PALSY

Defined as a persistent, but not necessarily unchanging, disorder of movement and posture due to a non-progressive disorder of the immature brain.

This excludes diagnoses such as brain tumours and spinal cord disease. The term implies that motor function is not simply delayed, but also follows a course that is not seen in the normal child. Prevalence is 2 per 1000 live births.

Causes of cerebral palsy

Prenatal

- Genetic forms – autosomal recessive and autosomal dominant
- Cerebral malformation
- Alcohol
- Substance abuse
- Infection (TORCH)
- Intra-uterine growth retardation

Perinatal

- Hypoxic ischaemic encephalopathy
- Ventricular haemorrhage
- Hypoglycaemia

Postnatal

- Meningitis
- Encephalitis
- Head injury

DIFFERENT TYPES OF CEREBRAL PALSY AND THEIR SPECIFIC PROBLEMS

Hemiplegia

This leads to varying degrees of spasticity in the affected side of the body, requiring physiotherapy to prevent the worst deformities developing. Weakness is usually more pronounced distally. The incidence of epilepsy and related disorders is related to cortical involvement – sensory defects, visual field defects and cranial nerve involvement should all be looked for.

Most children will walk by 18–24 months, if not other pathologies should be considered or the cerebral palsy extent reviewed. Splints may be used at night to prevent contractures. Special shoes help to equal leg lengths that may be discrepant due to limb shortening. Orthopaedic surgery has much to offer, with elongation of the Achilles tendon, although this is rarely required before 5 years of age.

Diplegia

In this situation the limbs on both sides of the body are affected, legs more than arms. More severely affected children never walk. It is more common in pre-term, low birth weight infants and in those who had an abnormal labour or delivery.

Quadriplegia

There is four limb and often bulbar involvement with the arms more severely affected than the legs. Initially young children are hypotonic with episodes of axial stiffening and extension. As they grow older the tone increases producing rigidity with pyramidal signs. The windswept hip deformity is particularly characteristic, the adducting hip being at risk of dislocation. Scoliosis can be severe and should be treated aggressively.

Bulbar muscles, usually spared in hemiplegia and diplegia, are commonly affected. Severe mental retardation and fits are common. Many affected infants are microcephalic.

Children with spastic quadriplegia have many problems and require a considerable multidisciplinary input usually co-ordinated through the local child development unit.

Surgery to relieve contractures is often performed.

Ataxic

Here the motor disorder is cerebellar ataxia, but this is usually associated with a diplegia. It is usually diagnosed relatively late – you need to reach a certain stage of development before cerebellar deficit is noticeable. It is difficult to diagnose and you must look for other causes of cerebellar dysfunction e.g. tumours and other progressive disorders (Friedreich's ataxia, ataxic telangiectasia, metachromatic leukodystrophy).

Athetoid

This involves involuntary movement of the limbs. Choreoathetosis is largely associated with hyperbilirubinaemia, the more severely disabled dystonic cases occur in severely asphyxiated term babies. The dystonic movements seen in the term asphyxiated infants involve slow movements with extension of the trunk and limbs. Other system involvement is common and should be looked for.

There are many children who fall into the category of mixed forms of cerebral palsy e.g. ataxia and diplegia. The importance is not in categorising their cerebral palsy but in determining the overall ability and disability of the child and working with that.

NOTES ON INVESTIGATION OF CEREBRAL PALSY

You may be asked how to investigate a child with cerebral palsy, clearly not all children with static cerebral palsy can be fully investigated, and this is usually reserved for those with

- the lack of an obvious cause e.g. hypoxic ischaemic encephalopathy
- loss of skills
- familial occurrence
- encephalopathy
- unusual features e.g. nystagmus
- lower motor neurone signs
- symmetrical signs

Useful investigations would include

- CT or MRI of head – MRI if neuronal migration defects were being considered
- Chromosome analysis
- Electroencephalogram
- Congenital infection screen
- Metabolic screen
- Ophthalmologic assessment
- Hearing tests
- Physiotherapy assessment

NOTES ON MANAGEMENT OF CEREBRAL PALSY

The treatment of cerebral palsy is something you may be expected to talk about at length and it is very important that you know all the aspects of management. This can arise, and commonly does, during any part of the exam.

Management involves a multidisciplinary approach, usually with the involvement of a child development unit. The team will consist of a:

Paediatrician

- Usually in a co-ordinating role

Physiotherapist

- Provides the greatest day-to-day contribution.
- Involved with the child from an early stage. Helps in preventing severe contractures and deformity as well as aiding as much normal motor development as possible

Communication therapist

- Involved early, providing help with feeding problems
- Later with speech
- Encourage parents to stimulate their children, and help them develop as much communication as possible, whether it be normal speech, sign language or a mixture of both

Occupational therapist

- Involved in adapting the environment to aid the child's functioning
- Involved in adapting play within the home to aid development.

Social worker

- Along with all the therapists having close links with the family
- Provides support for the family helping with periods of stress
- Arranging holidays and social admissions/respite care should the need arise

Others include

- Dietician; Educational pyschologist; Psychologist; Teacher; Ophthalmologist; Orthoptist; Audiologist; ENT surgeon; Orthopaedic surgeon.

CEREBRAL PALSY – CASES

These three cases are real and are meant to get you thinking about how to deal with and talk about children with cerebral palsy who you see in the exam. You need to make contact with whoever runs the child development unit in your area and arrange to see and discuss some cases.

Case 1 – 5-year-old boy

Peter is a thin boy who walks with a Trendelenburg positive gait, there is muscle wasting and decreased tone in the left leg. He has brisk reflexes with up-going planters and short tendo-achilles in the left side. No involvement of any other limb, particularly left arm normal.

Diagnosis – monoplegia involving the left leg

Discussion points
- What could be the cause?
- Why has he got a tight tendo-achilles on the affected side (contractures)?
- How would you treat his shortened achilles tendon (physiotherapy and surgery if necessary)?

Case 2 – 10-year-old girl

Jade is a thin looking girl with gross muscle wasting of all four limbs. She is lying in a windswept position (alternatively, she could be in a wheelchair with support). She is drooling. There is generalised hypertonia with contractures and increased reflexes. Both planters are up-going...

The diagnosis is spastic quadriplegia. I would like to examine the cranial nerves as she may have a pseudo-bulbar palsy.

Discussion points
- Multi-disciplinary care
- Feeding and nutritional status

Case 3 – 15-month-old boy

Joshua is thin. he has a spastic posture with minimal anti-gravity movement. He is drooling. I would like to examine his gross motor function, eyes and cranial nerves...

Discussion points

- Multi-disciplinary care
- Feeding and nutritional status
- How long do you think it takes to feed him lunch?
- How could his nutritional status be improved?
- What alternative methods of feeding could be used (gastrostomy)?
- What is the role of gastro-oesophageal reflux?

NEUROMUSCULAR DISEASE

This is another group of disorders which are seen with disproportionately high frequency in the exam and hence you need to know about them in considerable detail. These include diseases affecting the lower motor neurone either at the anterior horn cell, nerve fibre, neuromuscular junction or muscle. There are certain cases frequently seen in the exam. There are two main scenarios which we will deal with separately. The older child with neuromuscular disease and the floppy infant.

The older child

Commonly seen cases

- Duchenne muscular dystrophy
- Kugelberg-Welander disease
- Dermatomyositis
- Peroneal muscular atrophy

NOTES ON NEUROMUSCULAR DISEASE IN THE OLDER CHILD

DIFFERENTIAL DIAGNOSIS

Anterior horn cell

- Spinal muscular atrophy
- Poliomyelitis

Nerve fibre

- Infectious polyneuritis – Guillain-Barré syndrome
- Peroneal muscular atrophy
- Leukodystrophies
- Poisons

Neuromuscular junction

- Myasthenia gravis

Muscle

- Muscular dystrophy   Duchenne's
  Becker's
  Fascioscapulohumeral dystrophy
  Limb girdle dystrophy
- Dystrophia myotonica
- Inflammatory   Polymyositis, dermatomyositis
- Metabolic disease   glycogen storage disease
- Thyroid disease
- Steroids

NEUROMUSCULAR DISEASE IN THE OLDER CHILD: CASES

1. ANTERIOR HORN CELL

Spinal muscular atrophy type III (Kugelberg-Welander disease)

> **Case** – 14-year-old boy
>
> *Andrew is a thin looking boy who walks with a waddling gait. He has a positive Gower's sign. Examination of his peripheral nervous system shows reduced muscle bulk, hypotonia and absent tendon reflexes. There is a proximal muscle weakness. When his arms are outstretched, he has winging of the scapula and a fine tremor.*

The diagnosis is spinal muscular atrophy type III.

Notes

- Autosomal recessive
- Gene deletion known – diagnosis possible from the DNA
- Present age 5–15 with waddling gait/difficulty climbing stairs/ proximal muscle weakness
- Gower's positive
- Also – tongue fasciculation, reduced power (mostly proximal), reduced reflexes

Differential diagnosis

Limb girdle muscular dystrophy – see later

The two conditions have similar clinical features and are difficult to distinguish. This needs DNA analysis, electromyography and nerve conduction studies.

2. NERVE FIBRE

Guillain Barré Syndrome

> **Case** – 10-year-old girl
>
> *Jennifer is a well looking girl who is lying flat in bed. She has reduced tone in her lower limbs associated with depressed tendon reflexes and symmetrical weakness, which is more pronounced distally than proximally. I would also like to examine her cranial nerves and perform spirometry.*

The diagnosis is Guillain-Barré syndrome

Notes

- May get if there is a case on the ward in recovery phase
- It starts 10–14 days after a viral prodromal illness
- It is characterised by a symmetrical ascending flaccid paralysis
- Distal sensory loss or paraesthesia occur but are less marked than the motor symptoms and signs
- Examine for reduced tone and absent or reduced tendon reflexes
- Flexor plantar response
- Examine the cranial nerves as they are prone to ptosis and seventh nerve palsies
- The illness must be monitored with daily spirometry as the onset of respiratory failure is insidious and life threatening
- The main prognostic indicator is time to initial improvement after maximal weakness, those recovering after 16 days having a worse prognosis

NB Polio (unlikely to see but may get asked about) starts with an influenza type illness followed by muscle pain and then progressive ascending asymmetrical paralysis, worse in the legs.

Peroneal muscular atrophy

> **Case** – 12-year-old boy
>
> *Jordan is a 12-year-old boy who has pes cavus. There is associated weakness and wasting of the distal muscles of the leg, in particular he has weakness of foot dorsiflexion. His plantar response is down going. I would like to test the sensation in his feet.*

The diagnosis is peroneal muscular atrophy.

Notes

Also known as hereditary motor and sensory neuropathy type I, it usually begins in late childhood. The peroneal and tibial nerve are damaged, causing foot drop and the characteristic distal wasting. Sensory nerves conveying proprioception and vibration also become involved. The main differential diagnosis is Friedreich's ataxia, which is characterised by ataxia, Romberg's positivity, absent tendon reflexes and up-going plantars. Treatment is by stabilisation of the ankle joint with ankle-foot orthoses.

3. MUSCLE

Duchenne muscular dystrophy

> **Case** – 8-year-old boy
>
> *Samuel is an 8-year-old boy who is able to walk with the aid of a walking frame and foot orthoses. He has a wide based gait and an exaggerated lumbar lordosis. His calves are hypertrophied. On examination of the peripheral nervous system it is apparent he has a positive Gower's sign and reduced muscle bulk of his thighs, there is weakness of his hip flexors. There are absent knee jerks but brisk ankle jerks. I would like to examine his back for a scoliosis.*

The diagnosis is Duchenne muscular dystrophy

QUESTIONS

How do you confirm the diagnosis?
What is the differential diagnosis?
What is the prognosis?

NOTES ON DUCHENNE MUSCULAR DYSTROPHY

Incidence 1 in 3500 live born males. X-linked recessive. Gene locus known and is at Xp21. A third of cases represent a new mutation. Females may be symptomatic as a consequence of the random inactivation of one of the X chromosomes.

Usually present between the ages of 3 and 5 with delayed walking, waddling gait and difficulty with stairs. Calf muscle hypertrophy is often present. Most reflexes disappear early in the disease apart from the ankle jerk which disappears late.

Creatinine phosphokinase is usually abnormally high at birth and at diagnosis. Diagnosis is by DNA studies looking at the dystrophin gene. Electromyography and muscle biopsy can also be done, both of which show typical features. Complications arise from cardiac, respiratory and skeletal muscle involvement. Scoliosis is common. Physiotherapy input is important. The children need a wheelchair by the second decade. Prior to that a walking frame is used. Usually fatal during the second or third decade.

NOTES ON OTHER MUSCULAR DYSTROPHIES

Becker's muscular dystrophy

- Incidence is 1 in 30,000. Presents later than Duchenne muscular dystrophy. The gene defect is at the same locus as Duchenne muscular dystrophy. Cardiac and respiratory muscle involvement is rare. The creatinine phosphokinase is high at diagnosis. EMG and muscle biopsy are helpful in establishing a diagnosis. Dystrophin is abnormal.

Fascioscapulohumeral muscular dystrophy

- Facial and shoulder girdle muscles affected. The face is typically expressionless and there is also winging of the scapula, with shoulder muscle weakness.

Limb girdle muscular dystrophy

- Hips and shoulder muscles are affected and the condition progresses distally. Affected children can get calf muscle hypertrophy and ankle contractures which causes confusion with Becker's muscular dystrophy. Onset is in late childhood and most are wheelchair bound by age 30.

Dermatomyositis

- Covered in rheumatology chapter
- The asymmetry helps to distinguish it from other muscle disease e.g. limb girdle dystrophy

THE FLOPPY INFANT

Cases commonly seen in the exam

1. Werdnig-Hoffman disease
2. Myotonic dystrophy
3. Down's syndrome
4. Failure to thrive

Differential diagnosis

- You may see a hypotonic infant and be asked for a full differential diagnosis

It is important when reviewing the list to remember that there are many causes of the 'floppy infant' that can be seen in the exam and that both neurological and systemic conditions need to be considered. A full systematically organised differential diagnosis is listed.

Differential diagnosis of the floppy infant

Central

- Encephalopathy
- Intracranial haemorrhage
- Degenerative Disease e.g. infantile Gaucher's disease Neurometabolic disease e.g. Zellweger's

Spinal cord

- Spina bifida
- Transection of the cord e.g. following complicated breech delivery
- Haematoma
- Tumour

Anterior horn cell

- Spinal muscular atrophy (Werdnig-Hoffman disease)
- Poliomyelitis

Nerve fibre

- Demyelinating disease e.g. Guillain-Barré syndrome

Neuromuscular junction

- Transient neonatal myasthenia gravis

Case – 6-month-old girl

Samantha is a happy looking child who is visually alert. She is lying flat on her back with obvious paucity of movement and only minimal antigravity movement. She has a bell-shaped chest and paradoxical 'see-saw' respiration. When pulled to sit and on ventral suspension there is head lag and poor tone. She has no sitting posture. Tendon reflexes are absent.

Muscle

- Congenital myopathies
- Congenital myotonic dystrophy
- Congenital muscular dystrophies
- Pompe's disease

Systemic causes of hypotonia

In addition to those mentioned above:

- Trisomy 21
- Prader-Willi syndrome

Acute and chronic childhood illnesses can cause hypotonia particular examples include:

- Hypercalcaemia
- Renal tubular acidosis
- Rickets
- Hypothyroidism
- Coeliac disease
- Cystic fibrosis
- Failure to thrive

1. ANTERIOR HORN CELL

Werdnig Hoffman disease (Spinal Muscular Atrophy type one)
Diagnosis infantile spinal muscular atrophy

Discussion points
- Investigation and differential diagnosis
- Genetic counselling – gene probe available
- Care of the infant with a life threatening condition

Notes
- Autosomal recessive Chromosome 5
- Presents in the first year
- Watchful, alert, but immobile infant
- Frog-like posture, bell-shaped chest with see-saw respiration
- Muscle weakness, hypotonia, reduced or absent reflexes and fasciculation
- Life span 12–18 months
- Diagnosis is essentially a clinical one. Gene probe available.

2. MUSCLE

Myotonic dystrophy (dystrophica myotonica)

Myotonia is the failure of muscle to relax after contraction. Myotonic dystrophy is an autosomal dominant condition which shows genetic anticipation. The gene has been isolated to chromosome 19. The condition is characterised by progressive myotonic weakness particularly affecting the face, jaws, neck and distal muscles.

The early presentation is as the hypotonic floppy infant (= congenital myotonic dystrophy). The clue is the mother who is likely to have flat immobile face and myotonia (failure to relax) when you shake her hand.

Older child will present with a myotonic, flat immobile face, hypotonia, poor muscle bulk, weakness and reduced or normal reflexes. The extent of the motor defect is quite variable.

Congenital myotonic dystrophy

There is often a history of reduced fetal movements. The infant is floppy from birth – the myotonia presenting later. There is a facial diplegia with a triangular facies. There are often respiratory problems after birth. Associations in infancy include talipes and hip problems. The most severe form presenting in the neonatal period has a mortality of 75% in the first year.

In the majority of cases it is the mother who is affected but it can be the father. The investigation of choice is an EMG.

ATAXIA

Remember that ataxia can be due to a cerebellar or a dorsal column problem.

Common cases

1. Friedreich's ataxia
2. Ataxia telangiectasia
3. Ataxic cerebral palsy

DIFFERENTIAL DIAGNOSIS OF ATAXIA

Acute

- Infectious and post infectious e.g. chicken pox, mycoplasma measles
- Structural lesions e.g. tumours, hydrocephalus
- Toxic e.g. phenytoin, metabolic disorders
- Vascular e.g. basilar artery thrombosis

Intermittent

- Migraine
- Epilepsy
- Inherited recurrent ataxia (e.g. Hartnup disease)

Chronic ataxia

- Perinatally acquired e.g. hypoxic ischaemic encephalopathy
- Cerebellar malformation e.g. Dandy-Walker syndrome
- Spinocerebellar degeneration e.g. Friedreich's ataxia
- DNA repair abnormalities e.g. ataxia telangiectasia, xeroderma pigmentosa
- Metabolic e.g. Wilson's disease, leukodystrophies, abetalipoproteinaemia, Batten's disease
- Refsum's disease – phytanic acid storage disorder, peripheral neuropathy, deafness and retinitis pigmentosa
- Vitamin E deficiency – abetalipoproteinaemia
- Dysgenesis of the cerebellar vermis e.g. Joubert's syndrome

FRIEDREICH'S ATAXIA

= spinocerebellar degeneration

Case – 12-year-old boy

Peter is a well looking boy who on walking has an ataxic gait. He is Romberg's positive. He has pes cavus of his feet, up-going plantar responses and absent ankle jerks.

The diagnosis is Friedreich's ataxia, I would also like to examine his cardiovascular system.

Notes

This is a progressive ataxia with pyramidal tract dysfunction. Inheritance is usually autosomal recessive. The gene locus is on chromosome 9. It usually presents before the fifteenth birthday with loss of position and vibration sense. Other features include absent tendon reflexes, extensor plantars, sensory ataxia (positive Romberg's), nystagmus, pes cavus, kyphoscoliosis, cardiac abnormalities (hypertrophic cardiomyopathy) and an increased risk of diabetes mellitus. Treatment is largely supportive. Death is usually secondary to cardiac complications.

Older child ataxia plus positive Romberg's think Friedreich's ataxia

---

ATAXIA TELANGIECTASIA

This is an autosomal recessively inherited condition. The gene locus is on chromosome 11. The ataxia is cerebellar and usually presents in early childhood. The telangiectasia is characteristic and usually starts at age 5–6 years. The main areas initially are the bulbar conjunctiva and ears. A third of these children develop malignancy. There is an increased risk of recurrent infection with a low IgA and IgG. The alphafetoprotein is usually raised. There is a 50–100 fold greater chance of developing lymphoreticular malignancy as well as brain tumours.

SPINA BIFIDA

Case – 8-year-old boy

John is a well looking boy who is unable to walk alone and uses a wheelchair. He is wearing a nappy. Examination of his lower limbs reveals reduced muscle bulk proximally and distally. There is reduced power and tone in his legs and tendon reflexes are absent. I would like to examine his back...which reveals a healed surgical scar in the lumbosacral area and scoliosis.

The diagnosis is spina bifida.

Case – 3-year-old girl

Jessica is a well looking girl who is able to walk with the aid of calipers and a walking frame. She has a waddling gait and neurological signs consistent with a lower motor neurone lesion. Examination of her back reveals a surgical scar over the lumbar region. I would like to examine her for scoliosis and measure her head circumference...

The diagnosis is spina bifida.

Discussion points

- What associated problems might you expect?
- How do we attempt to prevent spina bifida?

NOTES ON SPINA BIFIDA

- Folic acid supplementation before conception and during the first trimester has been shown to reduce the risk of spina bifida.
- In all but the mildest sacral lesions there is some degree of hydrocephalus caused by a hind brain malformation. This is displacement of the fourth ventricle below the foramen magnum causing obstruction of the CSF as it tries to drain to the basal cisterns.

Associated problems to look for

- Hydrocephalus, offer to measure head circumference
- Joint contractures
- Scoliosis
- Ulcers on feet (sensory neuropathy)
- Incontinence of urine and faeces with patulous anus and palpable bladder
- Learning difficulties

NEUROCUTANEOUS SYNDROMES

These are uncommon in clinical practice but are commonly used as short cases in the exam. You need to know in detail the clinical signs and be able to discuss issues around each case.

1. Neurofibromatosis
2. Tuberous sclerosis
3. Sturge Weber syndrome
4. Incontenti pigmenti

1. NEUROFIBROMATOSIS

This is a very common and often quite straightforward short case.

INSTRUCTION

Examine this child's skin. What else would you like to examine?
Examine this child's eyes
Examine this child's gait. What else would you like to examine?
What is the inheritance pattern?
What renal complications may he get?

Case – 8-year-old boy

Simon has multiple café-au-lait spots with axillary freckling. His mother also has café-au-lait spots. I suspect the underlying diagnosis is neurofibromatosis type I.
I would like to examine...
I would like to check his mum...

Rest of examination

- Examine the visual fields for evidence of optic nerve gliomata which also cause proptosis and ptosis. Offer to examine the eye with a slit lamp for Lisch nodules
- Measure the blood pressure and listen for renal bruits
- Measure the head circumference (macrocephaly is common, hydrocephalus due to aqueduct stenosis is not)
- Examine the back for kyphoscoliosis

NOTES ON NEUROFIBROMATOSIS

Neurofibromatosis (1:4000)

Type II (10%) autosomal dominant inheritance, mostly new mutations, gene locus on chromosome 22.

Diagnosis

* Bilateral acoustic neuromas

or

* Unilateral acoustic neuroma and first degree relative with Neurofibromatosis type II

or

* Two of the following – neurofibroma, meningioma, glioma, schwannoma, juvenile posterior subscapular lenticular opacities

Type I (90%) autosomal dominant inheritance, 50% new mutations, gene locus on chromosome 17.

Diagnosed if two of the following features are present:

* Axillary or inguinal freckling
* Optic gliomas (15%)
* Distinctive osseous lesion e.g. kyphoscoliosis, tibial bowing
* Two or more neurofibromas or one plexiform neurofibroma
* Two or more Lisch (iris) nodules
* Prepubertal child 5 or more café-au-lait spots greater than 5 mm diameter
* Post pubertal 6 or more café-au-lait spots greater than 15 mm diameter
* A first degree relative with neurofibromatosis

2. TUBEROUS SCLEROSIS

This is usually introduced to candidates as the opportunity to examine the face of a child with adenoma sebaceum. These are warty lesions along the naso-labial folds but are not the earliest features, they appear in half of all patients by five years of age.

The earliest skin lesion is a depigmented macule which is leaf shaped and often difficult to see. Its appearance can be enhanced by use of a Wood's lamp.

A rare skin feature is the shagreen patch. Periungual fibromas are unusual in childhood so try to look at the parents' hands as you examine the child.

Case seen in the exam

- Child with shagreen patch and adenoma sebaceum
- What other features would you look for?
- Someone shown MRI head and kidney scans

NOTES ON TUBEROUS SCLEROSIS

Autosomal dominant inheritance with a 50% recurrence risk in offspring. 70% are new mutations. Prevalence in children is 1 in 10,000–15,000. Gene on chromosomes 9 and 11.

Seizures are common, often presenting as infantile spasms. All seizure types except petit mal have been described in tuberous sclerosis. Tuberous sclerosis is a cause of symptomatic epilepsy. The age of seizure onset and the severity of mental handicap are directly related, with most children in whom seizures develop under the age of two suffering mental handicap. Seizures respond well to anticonvulsants but rarely with complete seizure control. Vigabatrin is indicated, particularly in seizures associated with hypsarrhythmia on the EEG.

Prevalence of mental handicap is 30–50%.

Clinical features

- Skin   Hypopigmented macules
- Adenoma sebaceum present in 85% over the age of 5 years
- Periungual fibromas
- Shagreen patches
- Café-au-lait spots

- Teeth   Enamel hypoplasia
- Eyes   Choroidal hamartomas, retinal phakomas
- CNS   Cerebral astrocytoma, malignant glioma, hydrocephalus
- Kidney   Renal angiomas and polycystic kidneys
- Cardiac   Rhabdomyomas
- GI   Rectal polyp

Investigation

- Echocardiography
- SXR
- EEG
- CT
- MRI

Early death may occur due to seizures or tumours affecting the CNS, heart or kidney.

Adenoma Sebaceum 5 yrs.
ash-leaf spots   birth
Shagreen patch   - 2.5 yrs.
        (lumbosacral region)
Subungal fibroma - puberty

3. STURGE WEBER SYNDROME

In the exam you may see a child with a facial naevus. It is important if you do to know and be able to look for the associated CNS complications seen in some but not all children with a facial naevus.

Facial naevus (port wine stain)
- Present at birth = capillary haemangioma
- Sporadic
- Unilateral usually, but can be bilateral
- Upper face and eyelid but can be more extensive
- Glaucoma is an occasional complication

CNS
- Involvement of ipsilateral meninges and cortex
- Intracranial calcification
- Seizures
- Hemiparesis
- Mental retardation
- Not all have CNS complications

Investigation
- SXR intracranial calcification – rail track calcification seen by 2 years
- EEG, CT, MRI

Management
- Anti-epileptics
- Hemispherectomy/lobectomy occasionally considered as the epilepsy is very difficult to control
- Pulsed laser is used for the port wine stain

4. INCONTINENTI PIGMENTI

You will be presented with a girl with a very obvious rash which will be in the pigmented stage. You should offer to measure the head circumference and perform a full neurodevelopmental assessment as well as eye examination and ask the parent about seizure activity.

You may be asked about the inheritance as it is unusual:

- X-linked dominant
- Usually lethal in males

Clinical features

- Rash (present in neonatal period as an erythematous bullous rash which fades to pigmented lesions which are splashed across the skin as if by a paint brush)
- Seizures
- Mental retardation
- Spasticity
- Ocular abnormalities (benign mass in posterior chamber)

Hypomelanosis of Ito

This is a distinct syndrome with whorled, marbled areas of hypopigmentation. Half the children have neurological signs and symptoms. Most cases are sporadic.

YOUR NOTES

YOUR NOTES

YOUR NOTES

NOTES ON THE LONG CASE

The long case is an important part of the exam and a number of candidates fail on it. It is, however, if adequately prepared for, a part of the clinical exam in which you can perform well. Plenty of practice beforehand is therefore vital. Do this with a colleague or tutor. Practise seeing patients for the appropriate length of time. Practise presenting and think out and practise answers to questions on the case.

It is important to allocate your time carefully. The permitted time with the patient is 1 hour followed by 20 minutes with the examiner. You will need to spend some time establishing a rapport with the patient. It is essential that you take a very thorough history which should take about 20 minutes. This should be followed, during the next 15 minutes, by a careful physical examination that includes plotting the child's growth, checking blood pressure and testing the urine if appropriate. This will then give you about 20 minutes in which to collect your thoughts, to think about the case and to prepare the case for presentation to the examiners. You need to be prepared to present the case clearly and systematically, if possible from memory and in the way the examiner wants. You need to try to anticipate and think out the answers to the questions you may be asked or topics that the examiners may wish to discuss.

It is essential to practise all of this several times in order to become confident enough to do it well in the exam. Practising with a colleague who is doing the exam is helpful and motivating. It is also sensible to practise the long case presentation in front of a tutor who has done the exam.

The examiner will expect you to have clearly identified the patient's problems, to have a clear plan of management, including investigations, and an understanding of the social and domestic implications for the patient. You will also need to be able to identify the information which may need to be given to the patient and/or the relatives.

Much emphasis is made on the correct and problem orientated presentation. This really means presenting the patient clearly as one would do in a GP letter. The child may have active and inactive problems. The following pages contain examples of typical long case presentations.

EXAMPLES

Case One

I saw a 6-year-old girl with Down's syndrome. She has recently been diagnosed as hypothyroid. She is on treatment and well at the moment. Her other problems are:

- Obesity
- Constipation
- Previous surgery for Hirschsprung's disease
- Mental retardation
- Social

It may be that the entire discussion focuses on the mental retardation and how her schooling is sorted out:

- Pre-school learning support including portage
- Statement of special educational needs
- Review of special educational needs

Alternatively the examiner could focus on the medical complications seen in a child with Down's syndrome:

- Cardiac problems
- Hypothyroidism, other autoimmune problems
- Hirschsprung's disease
- Atlanto-axial instability
- Leukaemia

It is important to focus on all aspects of the long case, in particular the multidisciplinary aspects. It may be that you concentrate on just one area for a major part of the long case examination:

- How has the child's illness affected the parents and the other siblings? What has been the effect of the child's problems on the integrity of the family unit?

Children with cerebral palsy are often seen and in the same way the case must be presented in a systematic and organised way.

Case Two

I saw an 8-year-old boy with cerebral palsy. He has a spastic quadriplegia and is in a wheelchair. His main problems are:

- Difficulties with feeding, poor weight gain and recurrent chest infections
- Fits which are well controlled on anticonvulsant therapy
- Joint contractures and poor mobility
- Schooling
- Social

It may be that you then go on either to discuss the medical aspects of this child's care or the multidisciplinary management. It is important to remember this list.

Professionals involved in the Multidisciplinary Management of an 8-year-old with a spastic quadriplegia:

- Physiotherapist
- Occupational therapist
- Communication therapist
- Dietician
- Teacher
- Educational psychologist
- Social worker
- GP
- Community paediatrician
- Orthopaedic surgeon

This list would apply to many other potential long cases.

Case Three

I saw a 8-month-old child with bronchopulmonary dysplasia. His condition is stable at the moment. His main problems are:

- Chronic chest disease requiring home oxygen
- Severe failure to thrive – nasogastric tube feed dependant
- Pre-term – 25 weeks gestation
- Social problems

The subsequent discussion may focus on one or all of the above problems. Nutritional assessment will be of obvious concern and the reasons for his failure to thrive and the potential action that can be taken to overcome it may be discussed. Alternatively the social situation could be focused on with discussion about why there may be problems.

COMMONLY SEEN LONG CASES

Any condition may be seen and it is important not to be too put off if you don't know too much about the case you see. Keep your head and get as much information as you can, concentrating on putting the case together well and giving a well thought out multidisciplinary presentation. Remember, the child itself or accompanying parent will know a lot about the condition.

The following are examples of cases seen in the last few years:

- Cerebral palsy
- Ex premature baby with chronic lung disease
- Cystic Fibrosis
- Spina Bifida
- Down's syndrome
- Neurofibromatosis
- Crohn's disease
- Coeliac disease
- Nephrotic syndrome
- Chronic renal failure
- Ataxia telangiectasia
- Cyanotic congenital heart disease
- Marfan's syndrome
- Undiagnosed short stature
- Prader Willi syndrome
- Treacher Collins syndrome
- Atopy
- Noonan's syndrome
- Newly diagnosed diabetic
- Chronic asthma

Most of these conditions are covered elsewhere in the book but it is clearly essential to have a good knowledge of all of them. You will find it useful to think out the sorts of issues that may need discussion if you meet any of the above conditions as a long case.

NOTES ON THE VIVA EXAMINATION

The technique of the viva cannot be taught and it is a mistake to think that there is a standard answer to a particular question, particularly as subsequent questions will depend on your answers to the initial ones. It is important to give clear and precise answers and try to avoid creating the black hole which comes from discussing or listing as a differential diagnosis a condition that you know very little about. We have listed some commonly asked viva questions. The way to work through these is to think about (and practice the answer out loud) how you would answer the question if posed to you. It is advisable to prepare for such questions – talk about a paper you have read recently, talk about an ethical dilemma, discuss what audit is, discuss what evidence based medicine is.

It is wise to remember that anything can be asked in the viva. Credit should be given for sensible answers.

The question asked about the chosen topic is often vague and gives you the opportunity to lead the examiner towards the area of the subject about which you have most knowledge. For example 'Tell me about...', 'How would you manage...'. It is important to be prepared to be questioned in this way. The technique should be practised. The pitfall to this technique, which is why it doesn't always work, is that the examiner may be looking for a specific answer. He may, for example, discuss a particular resuscitation scenario and be looking for a particular answer. An example would be:

- A 4-day-old baby develops diarrhoea, what are your thoughts? The examiner is looking for primary lactose intolerance.

Practice questions in pairs. We have included many previously asked questions under the heading which represent the subgroups of the viva. Remember that there is no correct answer to any question. You might find it helpful, with a colleague, to ask each other questions and perhaps give each other the chance to talk for say 5 minutes on the topic.

Speak clearly and sensibly. Don't waffle. If you do not understand a question then say so.

Recently, examiners have been given a more structured framework within which to probe your knowledge and you will be expected to answer questions on:

- Basic sciences
- Emergencies
- Neonatal medicine
- Management of chronic illness
- Ethics
- Audit and research

Examples of commonly asked topics are given in the following pages.

BASIC SCIENCES

- Pathophysiology of Anaphylaxis
- Pathophysiology of diarrhoea
- Bilirubin metabolism and how phototherapy works – kernicterus and how it can be prevented. Why are > 50% of babies jaundiced?
- Pathogenesis of meningococcal septicaemia
- Describe the pathophysiological changes seen in infants post asphyxia
- How does the body maintain sodium homeostasis?
- Can you tell me anything about illness and superantigen disease?
- How does renal function in neonates evolve?
- Lung mechanics
- Pathogenesis of cystic fibrosis
- Nutritional content of milks/foods/supplements
- Describe the oxygen-dissociation curve. How is it different in infants?

EMERGENCIES

- Emergency collapse on the ward
- Management of diabetic ketoacidosis
- Management of acute asthma
- Management of status epilepticus
- Management of meningococcal septicaemia
- Management of hyperkalaemia
- Management of burns
- Management of coma
- Management of upper airway obstruction
- You are expecting a child to arrive in casualty in asystole, how would you prepare for this?

NEONATAL MEDICINE

- Management of collapse of a ventilated neonate
- Which blood vessels does the umbilical arterial catheter pass through?
- Management and investigation of ambiguous genitalia on the delivery suite
- Crash called to delivery suite for a flat baby – management
- How would you counsel an expectant mother who has had a child previously die of sudden infant death syndrome?
- Temperature control in neonates
- What may be done to reduce the vertical transmission of human immuno-deficiency virus?
- Be prepared to discuss neonatal screening for e.g. hypothyroidism
- How would you investigate and manage a baby born with cyanosis?
- What is the significance of a raised serum immuno-reactive trypsin on Guthrie testing? How would you investigate the baby further? (same question with phenylalanine)
- Give a differential diagnosis of neonatal hypoglycaemia
- What are the causes of neonatal apnoea? How do you treat it?
- How do you investigate and treat the infant of a drug abusing mother?
- Discuss the causes of macrosomia
- Why do we give vitamin K to newborn babies?
- How would you approach a 'floppy' baby?

MANAGEMENT OF CHRONIC ILLNESS

- Adolescent wards, transfer of children with chronic problems such as cystic fibrosis over to adult physicians
- Management of children with cerebral palsy
- How would you begin a consultation to tell a parent that their child has cystic fibrosis?
- How would you set up a paediatric diabetic outpatient unit at your hospital?
- Discuss the assessment of children with special educational needs.
- Discuss your outpatient management of a child with nephrotic syndrome
- How would you treat an 11 year old boy with nocturnal enuresis?
- Describe your management of a boy with chronic abdominal pain with no identifiable organic cause
- A toddler is referred to your clinic with a diagnosis of hyperactivity, describe your approach
- How do you manage chronic fatigue syndrome?
- Management of severe eczema in the outpatient setting
- Be prepared to discuss the most recent guidelines for asthma treatment
- What do you think is the role of play leaders on a paediatric ward?
- How would you assess a child referred to the clinic with headaches?
- What would you say to the mother of a child who has had their first febrile fit?
- A girl is referred to your clinic with Turner's syndrome. How would you manage her growth and puberty?
- How would you assess a 2 year old with unusual bruising?
- Describe your approach to a family with a 3 year old child newly diagnosed with peanut allergy.
- How do you manage an infant who is failing to thrive?
- Be prepared to talk at length about the investigation and treatment of urinary tract infections
- Talk about how you would investigate a child with frank haematuria

ETHICS

- Euthanasia and withdrawal of care (especially neonates and limits of viability)
- Choose your own ethical dilemma to talk about
- You are called to see a baby on the postnatal wards with probable Down's syndrome, what would you do?

AUDIT AND RESEARCH

- How would you look into asthma management in your hospital if you didn't think it was effective?
- List the constituents of an audit
- Tell me about a recent audit project that has altered your management of children
- What is the point of evidence-based medicine and is it practised ?
- Choose you own paper to talk about
- Choose a disease that is ideal for screening and explain why
- Do you know of any recent trials that have changed management – a good example is steroids and croup – how would you set up a trial to compare budesonide and oral dexamethasone?
- Tell me about screening, can use as an example phenylketonuria or primary hypothyroidism, how do you assess effectiveness. What are the criteria for a screening programme?
- Can use as an example phenylketonuria or primary hypothyroidism
- How to assess effectiveness
- Criteria for a screening programme
- How do you critically assess a paper when you read it?
- Know about basic statistic methods:
    - P values
    - Confidence intervals
    - Standard error/deviation
    - Correlation/regression
    - Student's t test

ARTICLES

Current Paediatrics

It is well worth going through copies of this journal which contains clear and concise reviews of paediatric topics which are at an appropriate level for the paediatric membership.

Archives of Disease in Childhood

Look through the last 2-3 years. In them there will be quite a number of papers that will help you with exam preparation. Current topics. Personal practice sections. Also look out a paper or two to discuss if asked to describe a paper that you have recently read.

Useful reviews and topical articles can also found in:

BMJ
Lancet
New England Journal of Medicine
Paediatrics
Journal of Paediatrics
Recent Advances In Paediatrics

GENERAL

RE Behrman et al, **Nelson Textbook of Paediatrics**, WB Saunders 1995

AGM Campbell & N McIntosh, **Forfar and Arneil's Textbook of Paediatrics**, Churchill Livingstone 1997

AEM Davies & AL Billson, **Key Topics in Paediatrics**, Bios Scientific Publishers 1998

T Stephenson & H Wallace, **Clinical Paediatrics for Postgraduate Examinations**, Churchill Livingstone 1995

AD Milner & D Hull, **Hospital Paediatrics**, Churchill Livingstone 1997

A Cade et al, **An Aid to the Paediatric MRCP viva**, Churchill Livingstone, 1995

CARDIOLOGY

N Archer & M Burch, **Paediatric Cardiology : An Introduction**, Chapman and Hall Medical 1998

CHILD ABUSE

CJ Hobbs et al, **Child Abuse and Neglect : A Clinician's handbook**, Churchill Livingstone 1998

COMMUNITY PAEDIATRICS AND CHILD DEVELOPMENT

RS Illingworth & V Dubowitz, **The Normal Child**, Churchill Livingstone 1991

L Polnay & D Hull, **Community Paediatrics**, Churchill Livingstone 1993

DMB Hall, **The Child with a Disability**, Blackwell Science 1995

DERMATOLOGY

J Harper & RS Wells, **Handbook of Paediatric Dermatology**, Butterworth-Heinemann 1990

EMERGENCIES

Advanced Life Support Group, **Advanced Paediatric Life Support**, British Medical Association 1997

ENDOCRINOLOGY

CGD Brook, **A Guide to the Practice of Paediatric Endocrinology**, Cambridge University Press 1993

GASTROENTEROLOGY

JA Walker-Smith & S Murch, **Diseases of the Small Intestine in Childhood**, ISIS Medical Media 1999

INFECTIOUS DISEASE

EG Davies et al, **Manual of Childhood Infections 2nd ed**, W B Sauders 1998

IMMUNISATION

Department of Health, **Immunisation against Infectious Disease**, The Stationery Office Books 1995

NEONATOLOGY

NRC Robertson, **A Manual of Neonatal Intensive Care**, Edward Arnold 1993

HW Taeusch & RA Ballard, **Avery's Diseases of the Newborn**, WB Saunders, 1998

NEPHROLOGY

RJ Postlethwaite, **Clinical Paediatric Nephrology**, Butterworth-Heinemann 1994

NEUROLOGY

R Appleton & J Gibbs, **Epilepsy in Childhood and Adolescence**, Martin Dunitz 1995

E M Brett, **Paediatric Neurology**, Churchill Livingstone 1996

V Dubowitz, **Muscle Disorders in Childhood**, W B Saunders 1995

PSYCHIATRY

ME Garralda, **Managing Children with Psychiatric Problems**, British Medical Journal Books 1993

RESPIRATORY

R Dinwiddie, **The Diagnosis and Management of Paediatric Respiratory Disease**, Churchill Livingstone 1997

V Chernick & TF Boat, **Kendig's Disorders of the Respiratory tract in children**, WB Saunders 1997

INDEX

PASTEST REVISION BOOKS

PasTest are the specialists in study guides and revision courses for professional medical qualifications. For 25 years we have been helping doctors to achieve their potential. The new PasTest range of books includes

MRCPCH Part 2 Paediatric Practice Papers: 2nd edition
This book offers 7 complete practice papers containing EEGs, ECGs and audiograms. Each Practice exam comprises 5 case histories and 10 data interpretations. Answers and detailed teaching notes are provided.

P Gringras, D Pal & M Greenberg   **ISBN: 1 901198 26 X**

Data Interpretation for the MRCP: Revised edition
10 data interpretation practice papers with strong clinical orientation. This book provides a wide selection of data and charts reflecting the demands of the exam.

P Clark & R Neilson   **ISBN: 1 901198 13 8**

Radiology for MRCP: 101 Cases with Discussion
This book incorporates a collection of radiological plates and discussion points for the aspiring candidate. Contains X-rays, MRI scans and CT scans with a section on understanding the principles of interpretation.

S Howling & P Jenkins   **ISBN: 1 901198 83 5**

To order any of the above titles, please contact PasTest on Freephone

0800 980 9814

PasTest, FREEPOST, Knutsford, Cheshire, WA16 7BR
Fax: 01565 650264 E-mail: books@pastest.co.uk
Web site: http://www.pastest.co.uk

PASTEST REVISION COURSES

PasTest is dedicated to helping doctors pass their professional examinations. We have over 25 years of specialist experience in medical education and over 4000 doctors attend our revision courses each year.

Experienced lecturers:
Many of our lecturers are also examiners who teach in a lively and interesting way to ensure you:

- are familiar with current trends in exams
- receive essential advice on exam technique
- are taught how to avoid the common pitfalls
- have plenty of mock exam practice

Outstanding accelerated learning:
Our up-to-date comprehensive course material includes hundreds of sample questions similiar to those you will experience in the exam. You will also receive detailed explanations, including charts and diagrams.

Choice of Courses:
PasTest has developed a wide range of high quality courses in various cities around the UK.

Don't take our word for it - here's what candidates say about our courses:

'It helped me to streamline my revision studies. Thank you very much!'
Dr Lahoti, Sheffield

'Absolutely brilliant – I would not have passed without it!! Thank you!'
Dr Rajapakse, London

'Thorough, extremely well prepared – I highly recommend it. Excellent'
Dr Gordon, Southampton

'Very methodically conducted revision and exam oriented course. I strongly recommend this for any exam goer!' **Dr Ramanujachar, Swansea**

'I felt the course was excellent value for money and I would (and do) recommend it to anyone!' **Dr Shawcross, Surrey**

For further details 'phone PasTest on:

Freephone 0800 980 9814

gço + b4c + Lещ∧